Surgical Anatomy of the Colon, Rectum and Anal Canal

Surgical Anatomy of the

Foreword by

ALEXANDER BRUNSCHWIG, M.S., M.D., F.A.C.S.

Attending Surgeon, Memorial Hospital for Cancer and Allied Diseases; Professor of Clinical Surgery, Cornell Medical School.

With Contributions by

TEODORO P. NUGUID, B.S., M.D., M.S.

Chief Resident in Proctologic Surgery, Temple University Medical Center

PHILADELPHIA • MONTREAL

Colon, Rectum and Anal Canal

HARRY E. BACON,
M.D., SC.D., LL.D., F.A.C.S., F.R.S.M. (Hon.), F.P.C.S. (Hon.)

Professor and Head, Department of Proctologic Surgery, Temple University Medical Center; Diplomate American Board of Surgery and of American Board of Colon and Rectal Surgery.

AND

PORFIRIO MAYO RECIO,
M.D., M.SC., F.P.C.S., F.I.C.S., F.A.C.S., F.P.C.G.

Assistant Professor of Surgery, College of Medicine, University of the Philippines, Attending Surgeon Philippine General Hospital and Hospital de San Juan de Dios; Diplomate American Board of Colon and Rectal Surgery; Secretary Philippine College of Surgeons.

69 *Illustrations*

J. B. LIPPINCOTT COMPANY

Distributed in Great Britain by
Pitman Medical Publishing Co., Limited, London

Library of Congress Catalog Card No. 62-8090

Printed in the United States of America

TO

ALEXANDER BRUNSCHWIG

In profound admiration for his prodigious energy and talent, for his vision, immense capacity for productive work, his leadership in surgical life—we dedicate this small volume for one whom we esteem affectionately for his humaneness and courageous devotion to the ideals of democracy.

Foreword

A comprehensive knowledge of anatomy is necessary for the proper execution of surgical procedures. This truism has been accepted down through the ages during which surgery has evolved from crude practice limited to the immediate care of traumas and simple incisions for the drainage of suppuration, to the present time where operations within the body cavities are performed with deliberation after elaborate preparations, and the use of all pertinent ancillary resources. At this time of great emphasis upon the physiologic and biochemical aspects of disease in the teaching of students and in medical writing there is scant attention paid to such a relatively static science as gross anatomy. It would appear that this area of medicine is taken for granted. From the point of view of advancing the frontiers of medical knowledge this is permissible. From the pedagogical point of view anatomy can hardly be neglected. The teachers of anatomy in the early modern eras were for the most part active clinicians and until not so long ago the budding surgeons teaching responsibilities in anatomy as preparation for surgery. This custom has been discontinued, and in the interest of maintaining a high level of performance of operative surgery, it is to be regretted.

Dr. Bacon, a distinguished surgeon and one who has devoted practically his whole professional career to the surgery of the colon, rectum, and anal canal, and Dr. Recio, are two of the outstanding authorities today in this field of specialization both in the United States and abroad. They have given the medical profession an excellent and authoritative work on the anatomy of the colon, rectum, and anal canal, presented in the traditions of the master surgeons of previous epoques, i.e., from the standpoint of the operating surgeon who is ever mindful of the necessity of anatomical knowledge to perform his operation with the highest degree of proficiency. Included in the discussions are pertinent references to the embryology and physiology of the colon and discussions of the anatomy of related structures, such as the ureters, peritoneal fossae, etc., which are of importance in operations upon the colon itself, as well as clinical anatomical aspects of the subject such as proctoscopic appearances of the lower large bowel.

The edition of this work is timely since there appears to be in process of evolution a special interest in pelvic surgery as a whole. This interest includes not only specialists in colon surgery but also urologists, gynecologists, as well as general surgeons. Diseases involving pelvic structures are oblivious of man made demarcations of surgical practice and may involve any or all portions of the pelvic contents of which the sigmoid, rectum, and anal canal are important components. Thus, an excellent work on the anatomy of the latter structures is a most welcome and important contribution, especially since it comes from such an authoritative source as these authors.

ALEXANDER BRUNSCHWIG, M.D.

Introduction

There is a sustained and increasing interest in the study of diseases of the colon, rectum and anal canal especially as regards surgical application. The number of surgeons who devote their time and practice or the greater part of their practice to surgery of the large bowel has increased immeasurably.

It has been a fortunate circumstance to have taught anatomy, operative surgery and proctologic surgery at Temple and at the Graduate School of the University of Pennsylvania to both undergraduate and postgraduate students during the past two and a half decades because in a large measure the present treatise represents an expansion of the material and experience of the authors. On repeated occasions the wide gap between freshman dissection, junior lecture and resident operative surgery has been evident. For this reason it has been the purpose of this discussion to provide a broad basic review on one hand with detailed surgical application on the other. The presentation of surgical anatomy of the colon, rectum and anal canal is an attempt on our part to offer a practical guide to, as well as provide a summary of current knowledge of, the anatomy and physiology of these regions. The fundamental data have been taken from numerous source books on anatomy and proctologic surgery. Pertinent investigations have been incorporated. Our published and unpublished investigations and experiments from the dissecting and operating tables and the morgue have been included. If the dilemma of the neophyte medico can be met and resolved and the avidity of the graduate students for additional knowledge satisfied in these pages, the sincere desire of the authors will have been fulfilled.

The authors would be ungrateful indeed if they did not express their profound appreciation to Dr. Teodoro P. Nuguid, our Chief Resident in proctologic surgery, who dedicated himself to the task of arranging and clarifying construction throughout the text. His assiduous application to detail and his patience in reviewing all descriptive data and references have proved of invaluable aid. Upon the return of our medical artist to Japan, numerous corrections were required in the illustrative material and, while minor in character, proved time-consuming and onerous. To this task Dr. Nuguid devoted himself and in addition read the proof with meticulous care.

The writers are indebted to Mr. Tetsuo Yajima, Head of the Department of Medical Art at the University of Chiba, Japan, for the excellence of the illustrations. For the loan of this brilliant medical artist we are grateful to our friend and colleague, the Professor of Surgery at the University, Doctor Komei Nakayama.

Without the able assistance of Miss Lucile Grebenc, consultant-editor in our department, whose experience and skill have contributed materially to the completion of this monograph, the preparation of this volume would have been protracted. Expressions of gratitude go to our secretaries, Mrs. Eva S. Recio and Miss Irene Engard for patiently typing the manuscript through several rewritings and to our understanding wives whose inspiration sustained us throughout.

Finally, we wish to thank the officers and personnel of the publishers, J. B. Lippincott Company, particularly Mr. Walter Kahoe and Mr. Brooks Stewart, for their counsel, co-operation and patience.

HARRY E. BACON, M.D.
PORFIRIO M. RECIO, M.D.

Contents

Chapter 1

Surgical Anatomy of Colon, Rectum and Anal Canal

The large bowel is that segment of the intestinal tract that is derived from the postarterial midgut, the hindgut and the proctodeal pouch. Hence, it extends from the cecoappendiceal region down to the anal opening. The large intestine has been variously subdivided into different anatomic and surgical segments. Its component parts include:

1. Cecoappendiceal region
   A. Vermiform appendix
   B. Cecum
2. Ascending colon
3. Hepatic or right colic flexure
4. Transverse colon
5. Splenic or left colic flexure
6. Descending colon
   A. Lumbar portion
   B. Iliac portion
7. Pelvic or sigmoid colon
8. Rectum
9. Anal canal

The term "colon" is generally reserved for the intraperitoneal portion of the large intestine, although some surgeons would even consider the cecum, and especially the appendix, as separate from the colon. Surgical experience has sanctioned the consideration of the terminal ileum with the cecum and has integrated the two parts into a common ileocecal region. The vermiform appendix, though an evagination of the cecal wall embryologically, is from the clinical point of view considered separate from the large bowel. Clinicians have divided the colon into a right hemicolon, extending from the cecoappendiceal region to the midtransverse colon or even a little beyond, and a left hemicolon, extending from the midtransverse colon to the rectosigmoid region. The right hemicolon, located in the right half of the abdominal cavity, is derived from the postarterial midgut, is supplied and drained by the superior mesenteric vessels and innervated by the vagus. It is primarily concerned with absorption. The left hemicolon, disposed in the left half of the abdominal cavity, is derived from the hindgut, is supplied and drained by the inferior mesenteric vessels and innervated by the sacral parasympathetics. It is primarily concerned with the storage and the expulsion of feces. The rectoanal tract was once considered as a separate surgical unit, but recent trends in surgical practice tend to combine the study and the surgery of the anal canal and the rectum with the study and the surgery of the colon.

EMBRYOLOGY OF COLON, RECTUM AND ANAL CANAL

Colon

The 3 layers of the embryo contribute to the formation of the colon, the rectum and the anal canal. The anal canal is derived from the ectoderm, while the remainder of the digestive tube is derived from the entoderm and the mesoderm. The entoderm forms only the mucous membrane and the numerous glands that line the colon and the rectum. The mesoderm develops into the peritoneum (somatic mesoderm) and the muscular and serosal coats of the bowel wall, and the vascular and connective tissues that later develop in these layers (splanchnic mesoderm).

The primitive gut develops from that portion of the yolk sac enclosed within the embryo. With incurvation of both ends to form the head and the tail folds of the embryo, the yolk sac becomes divided into 3 contiguous parts, depending upon the relation to the yolk stalk. These parts are (1) foregut—cranial to the yolk stalk, (2) midgut—at the region of the yolk stalk and communicating by way of the vitellino-intestinal tract with the yolk sac and (3) hindgut—caudal to the yolk stalk. Each of these divisions is supplied later by a branch from the dorsal aorta, coursing in the corresponding dorsal mesentery.

The communication between the yolk sac and the midgut becomes narrower as the yolk sac develops, becoming attenuated finally as a vitellino-intestinal duct in the yolk stalk with the separation of the embryo from the yolk sac. The primitive digestive tube or mesenteron is thus formed, appearing as a closed straight tube suspended in the mid-line of the body by a double-layered membranous sheet of mesoblast—the primitive mesentery. This mesentery has a ventral and a dorsal component which attach the primitive digestive tube to the corresponding body wall. In the course of subsequent development almost the entire ventral mesentery undergoes fusion and absorption, leaving the dorsal mesentery to fix the gut to the dor-

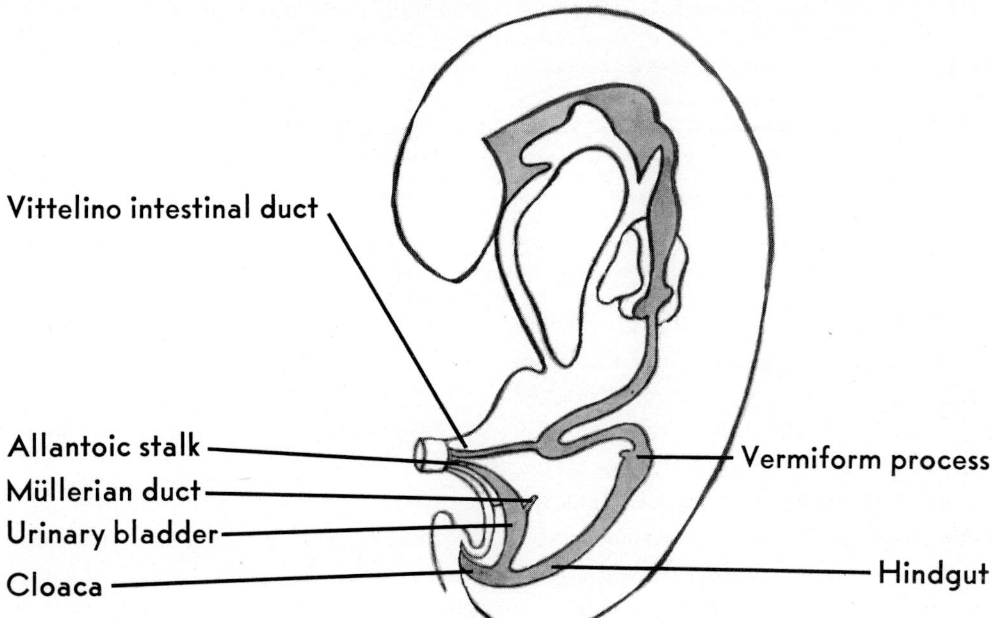

FIG. 1. Digestive tract of an embryo of 7.5 mm. Vermiform process is a dilatation of the lower intestinal loop that marks the boundary between the small intestine above and the large intestine below.

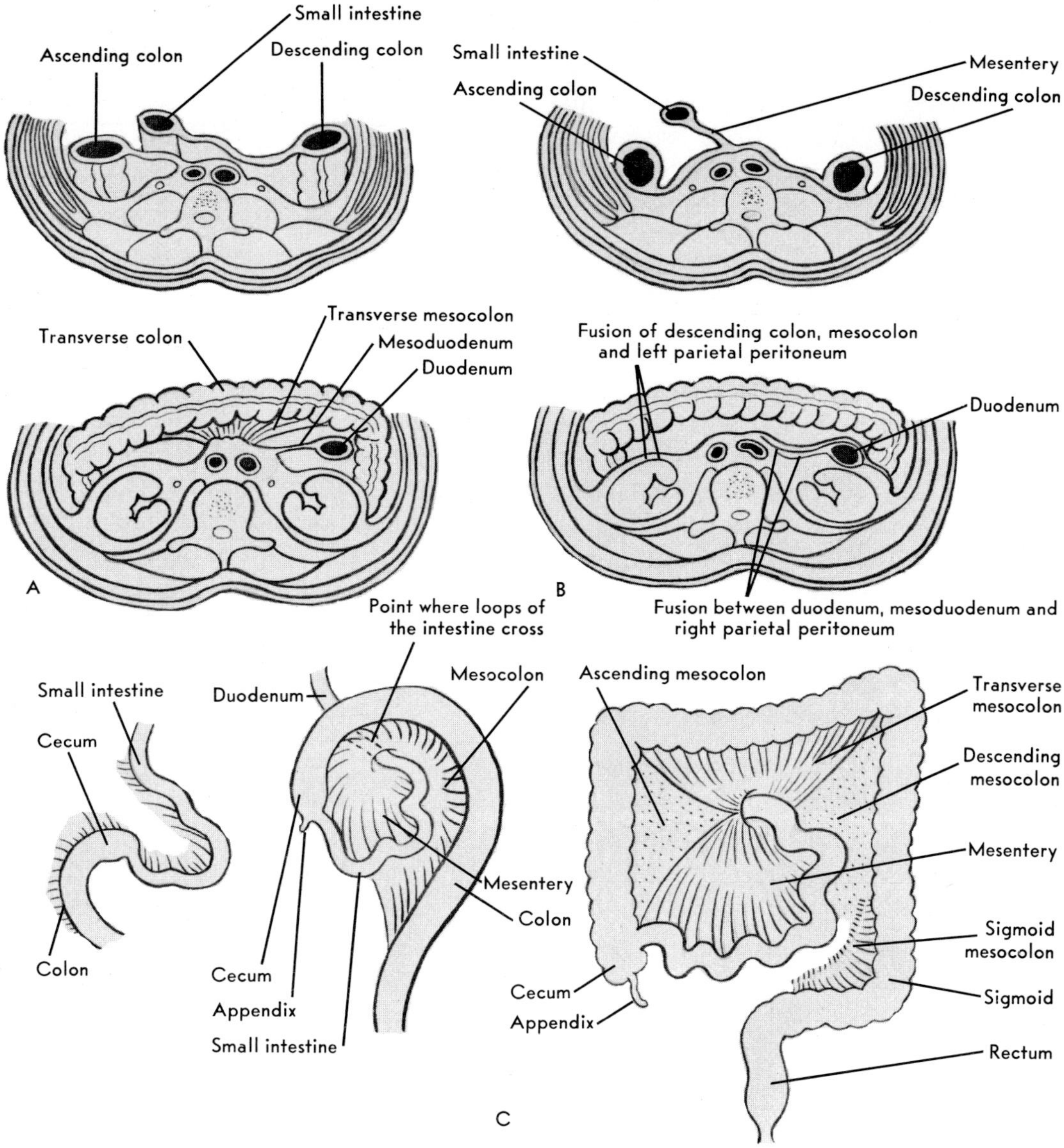

FIG. 2. Embryology of the large bowel. (A) Before posterior fixation. (B) After posterior fixation. (C) Rotation of the large bowel.

sal body wall. All the mesenteries normally found in adult life are derived from the dorsal mesentery.

The endodermal layer proliferates more rapidly than the developing mesoderm, with the result that the cavity is obliterated, and the tube is transformed into a solid cord of cells at the age of 4 to 8 weeks. Epithelial occlusion follows, resulting in isolated spaces which subsequently coalesce with one another, finally recanalizing the gut, which normally develops into a tube communicating at both ends with the outside.

Owing to the early fusion of the respective dorsal mesenteries to the dorsal body wall, the foregut and the hindgut become relatively fixed structures early in their development and thus show no loops in the adult form, where they remain mostly in the mid-line. With the arching of the body of the embryo, the midgut forms a convex loop owing to its mesenteric attachment to the dorsal body wall. The blood supply of the midgut develops from those of the yolk sac, the two vitelline arteries uniting to form a common trunk—the superior mesenteric artery. The segment of the midgut cranial to its vascular supply is called prearterial segment, with its arterial supply running up the prearterial mesentery, which later develops into the small bowel. The segment of the midgut distal to the superior mesenteric artery is called postarterial segment; it has its arteries running downward in the postarterial mesentery; later it develops into the right hemicolon.

During the age of 4 to 5 weeks, at the time of rapid endodermal proliferation, the midgut grows very rapidly, probably because it is relatively free, unlike the fixed head and tail ends of the gut. Thus, the embryonic coelom proper could not accommodate the rapidly lengthening bowel with its numerous loops in the process of being formed, and a portion of the midgut must be extruded through the narrow umbilical channel to the more capacious extraembryonic cavity of the umbilical cord. This results in a temporary physiologic herniation.

First Stage of Rotation. Preliminary rotation of the midgut loop occurs around the arterial axis until about the 10th week, when the rate of growth of the intra-embryonic coelom parallels that of the midgut loop which is simultaneously being recanalized. The omphalomesenteric or vitellino-intestinal vessel and duct becomes obliterated and contracts; when the cavity of the umbilical cord becomes similarly obliterated, the extruded midgut returns into the intra-embryonic coelom, thus spontaneously reducing the physiologic herniation. This reduction of the herniation is also helped by the contraction of the fibromuscular tissue about the superior mesenteric artery and the reduction in size of the liver. There is an orderly return of the small bowel loops so that the more distal loops are deposited caudally and to the right.

Second Stage of Rotation. The postarterial midgut is rotated more definitely in such a manner that the developing cecum lies under the right lobe of the liver, and the transverse colon is across the root of the superior mesenteric artery.

Third Stage of Rotation. Further rotation about the superior mesenteric artery occurs so that the cecum descends along the right flank, and the dorsal mesentery becomes fused to the posterior body wall, obliterating the mesentery of the cecum, the ascending colon, the hepatic flexure and the descending colon.

Rectum and Anal Canal

The development of the distal end of the digestive tube is closely related to that of the external genital apparatus. Even before there is formation of the head and tail folds, a small allanto-enteric diverticulum buds from the caudal wall of the yolk sac and grows into the loose mesenchymal tissue of the connecting stalk. As the tail fold bends and the hindgut is formed, and with further development of the connecting stalk, this allanto-enteric diverticulum is rotated so that it seems to migrate to the ventral aspect of the hindgut, while the distal part which is in the body stalk remains as the allantois. A saccular dilation appears at the subterminal portion of the hindgut caudal to the at-

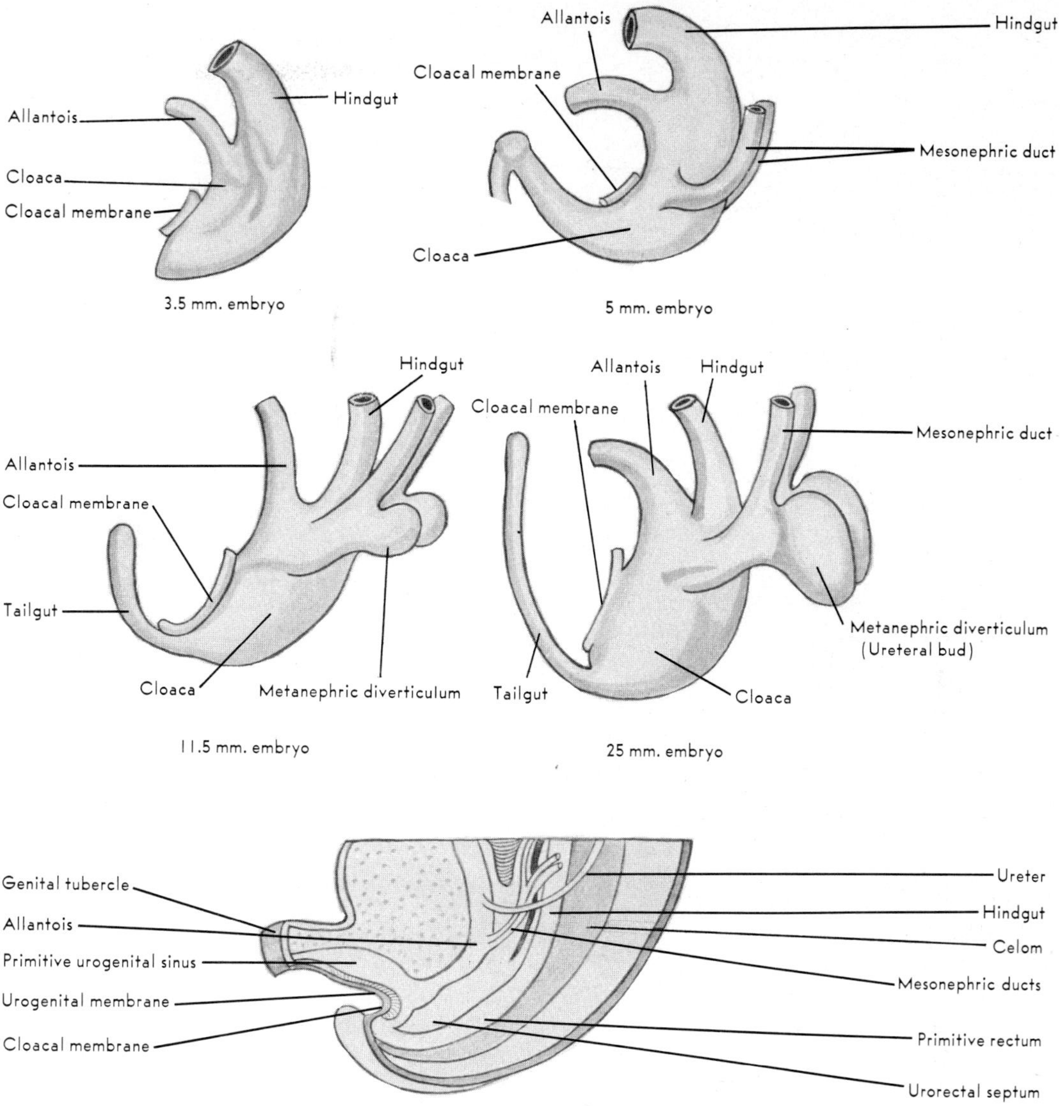

FIG. 3. Models of developing urogenital sinus; development and fate of cloaca.

tachment of the allantois and merges with the proximal end of the allanto-enteric diverticulum to form the cloaca. The cloaca is separated from the outside by fusion of ectoderm and entoderm, called the cloacal membrane. The terminal narrowed portion of the hindgut distal to the cloaca is called the tail gut (postanal gut), located as it is in the tail of the embryo. As the subterminal portion of the gut dilates in the 4 to 5 mm. embryo, it is joined by the common excretory duct (pronephric and mesonephric ducts) at the junction of the middle and the anterior thirds, and thus the common cavity formed is properly called the primitive cloaca. This primitive cloaca undergoes unequal expansion, elongating sagitally and flattening from side to side.

In the 5-mm. embryo, a cresentic vertical urorectal fold develops at each lateral cloacal wall, between the angle of the

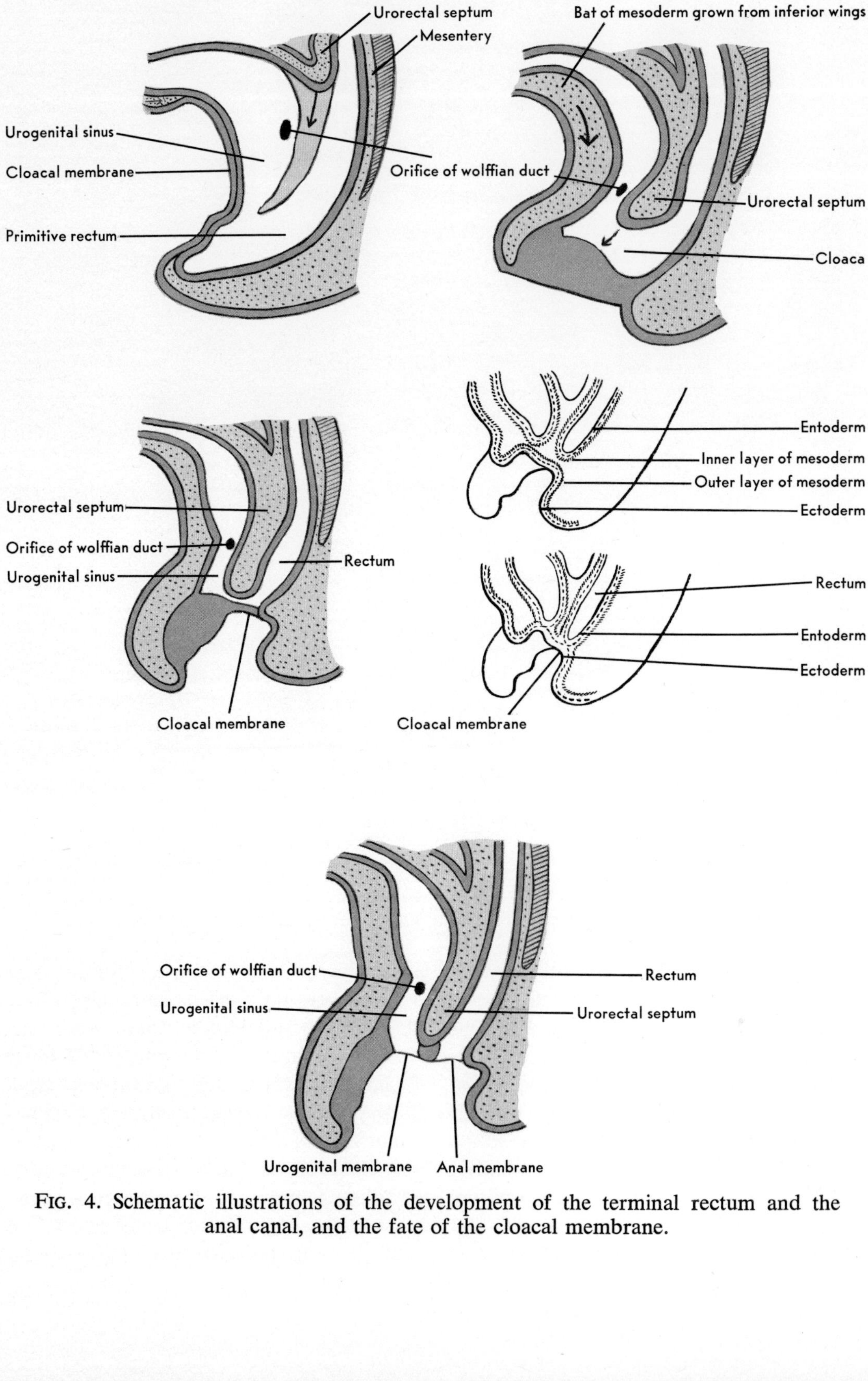

FIG. 4. Schematic illustrations of the development of the terminal rectum and the anal canal, and the fate of the cloacal membrane.

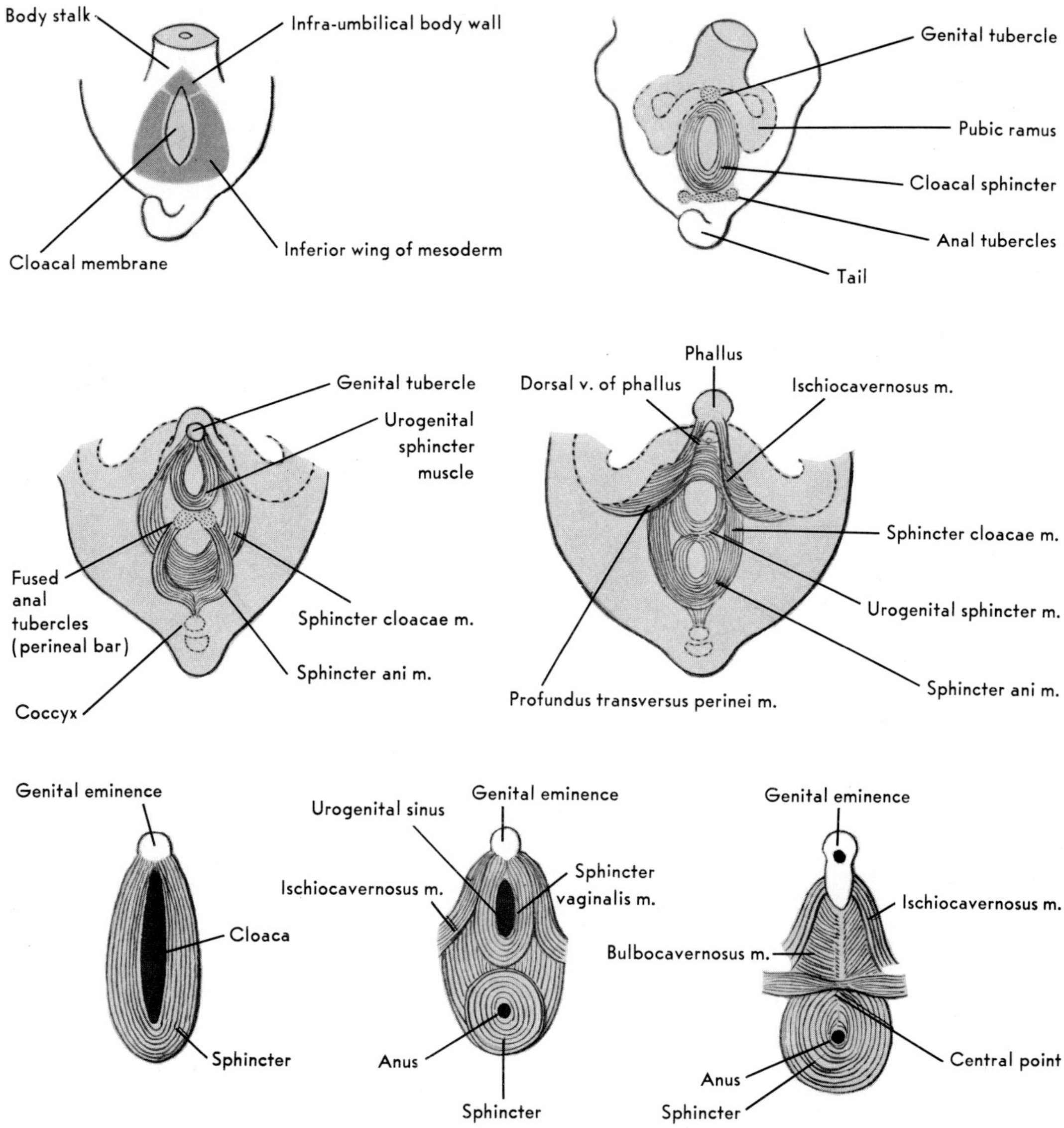

FIG. 5. Embryology. Evolution of perineal musculature.

allantois and the hindgut—Rathke's urorectal bar. This grows toward the mid-line and also descends toward the cloacal membrane. Later in the 8-mm. embryo, the cloacal cavity becomes divided by the growing urorectal bar into a smaller, dorsal, primitive rectum and a larger, ventral, primitive urogenital sinus connected by a cloacal passage between them. At this time, the latter part of the 6th week, mesoderm develops at the base of the body stalk, raising the ectoderm into genital swellings between which is a depression of the ectodermal layers of the cloacal membrane called primitive proctodeum, the site of the future anus. The descending primitive rectovesical (urorectal) septum fuses with the endodermal layer of the

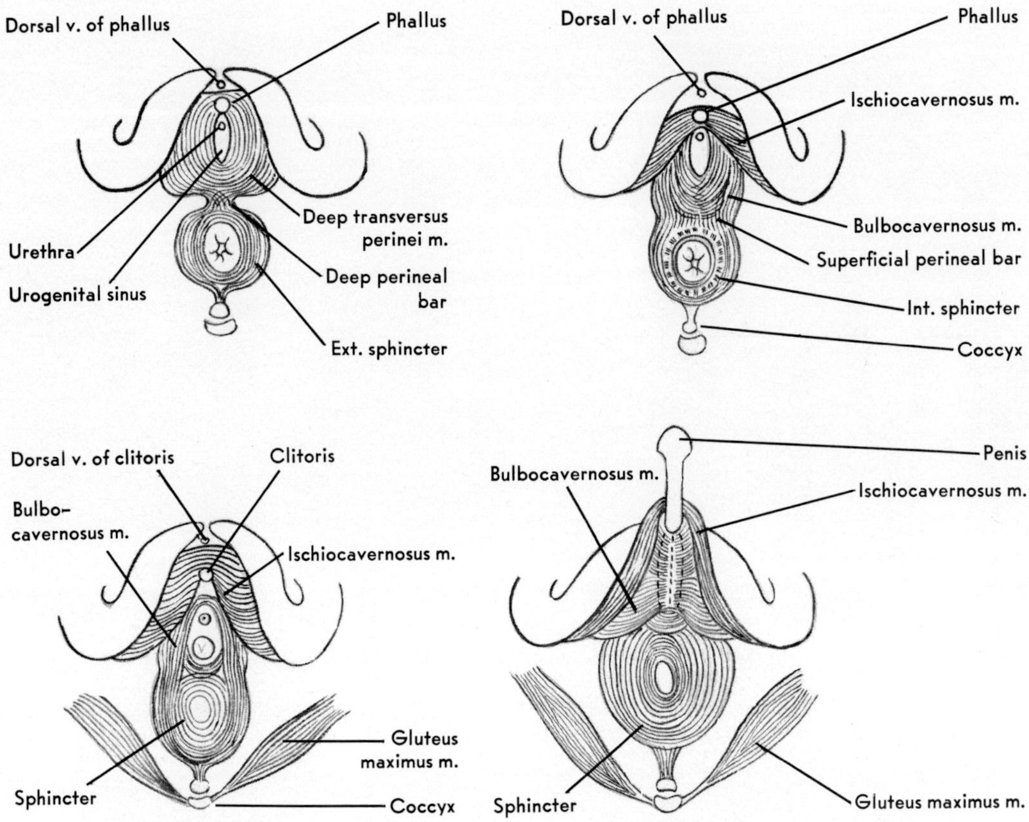

FIG. 6. Embryology. Demonstration of perineal and anal musculature.

cloacal membrane (16-mm. embryo, 6½ weeks), forming the primitive perineum. This primitive perineum is thus divided by the rectovesical septum into an anterior urogenital membrane, which later becomes the urogenital sinus, and a posterior anal membrane. During the development of the urorectal septum, the cloacal membrane is rotated so that instead of facing the anterior abdominal wall, it faces inferoposteriorly, due to regression of the tail and development of the infra-umbilical anterior wall.

The rising mesoderm transforms the proctodeal depression on the cloacal membrane into a funnel-shaped proctodeal pit which grows deeper into the tail end and finally fuses with the descending postallantoic gut to form the proctodeal plate or the anal membrane. At about the same time as the cloacal passage or duct is being obliterated, the tail gut or postanal gut is gradually being absorbed, even as the postallantoic gut descends. The future rectum develops as a spindle-shaped segment at the distal end of the postallantoic gut. It consists of an upper narrower part, the supra-ampullary portion, and a lower wider part, the ampulla. Because the descending postallantoic gut has a larger caliber, it has to adapt itself to the smaller proctodeal pit, and the former is even partially telescoped into the latter, due to the developing internal sphincter. This inequality in size of the lumen results in a drawstringlike effect, causing an internal

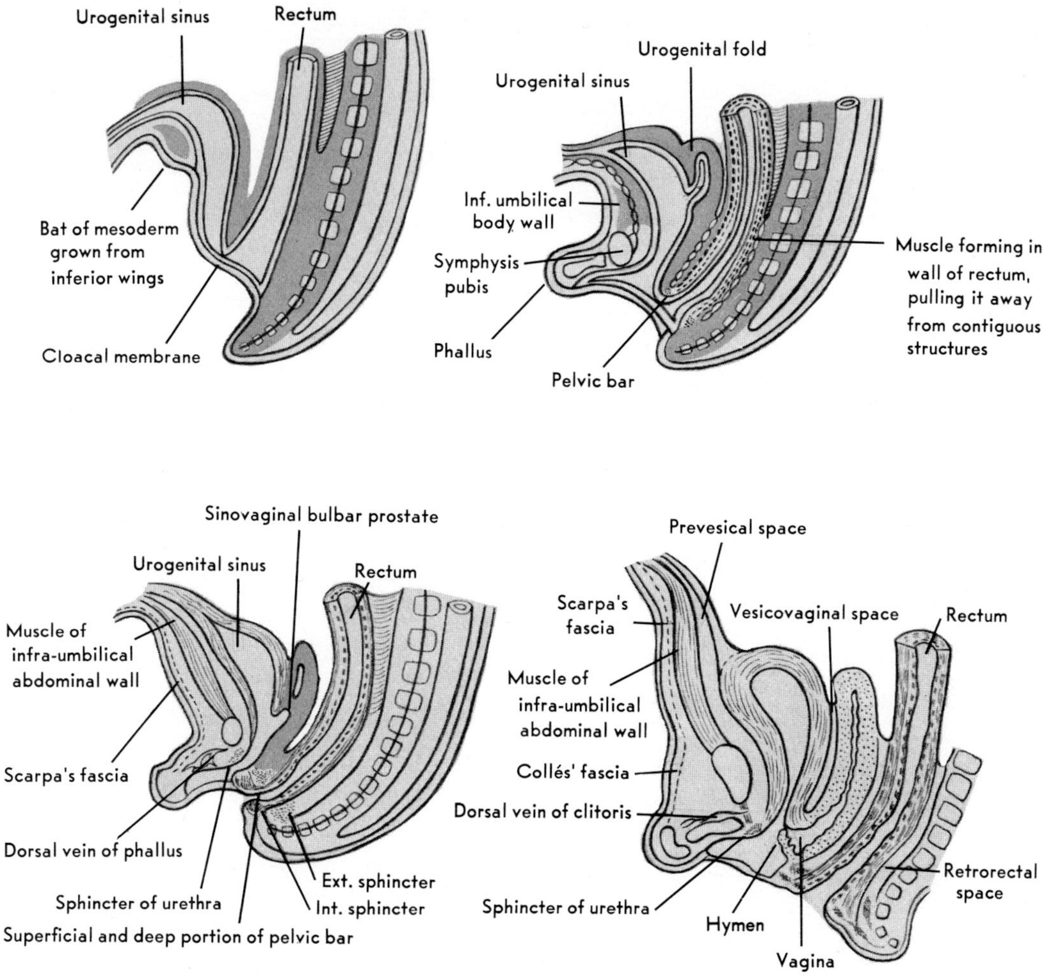

FIG. 7. Sagittal section of the caudal embryo. Note the separation of the common cloaca by the urogenital septum or pelvic bar to form the urogenital sinus anteriorly and the rectum posteriorly.

pleating of the rectal wall. Later, in the 9th week, in the 30-mm. embryo, the anal plate starts to disintegrate, and by the 12th week the anal membrane is completely disintegrated or absorbed, with the result that the rectum communicates with the exterior. The vestiges of the anal membrane are the conical teatlike anal papillae of Morgagni found punctuating the anorectal line. By the time the anal membrane ruptures, meconium has formed. It is a sterile, dark-green, mucilaginous material composed of secretion of intestinal glands, liver and pancreas, mixed with swallowed amniotic fluid, hair, vernix caseosa and desquamated cells from the intestinal epithelium.

In the female, the posterior wall of the urogenital sinus develops in conjunction with the uterovaginal canal, which results from the fusion of the lower portions of the müllerian paramesonephric ducts. Thus, any abnormal connection previously existing between the urogenital sinus and the descending postallantoic gut necessarily involves the vaginal wall.

CLINICAL SIGNIFICANCE AND SURGICAL CONSIDERATIONS

The foregoing embryologic discussion would be merely academic if it were of no clinical significance. As the colorectoanal tract is derived from all germ layers, almost any type of new growth may be encountered anywhere along its course from the cecum to the anal canal. Adenocarcinoma is found only in the colon and the rectum because the glandular lining of these segments develops from the entoderm. There has been an occasional exception to this rule. Epidermoid carcinoma can arise from the anal canal alone, since it develops from the ectoderm. More recent reports in the literature reveal that epidermoid carcinomas have been found also in the rectum and the rectosigmoid. This occurrence has been explained on the ground that (1) they may originate from embryonic cell rests, (2) they may originate from undifferentiated basal cells of the mucosa, (3) they may result from metaplasia of the superficial cells of the rectal mucosa, and (4) they may arise from anal ducts that have extended cephalad. The mesodermal or mesenchymal tumors as hemangioma, leiomyoma, lipoma, fibroma and hemangiopericytoma and the various sarcomas can develop from the portion of the bowel derived from the mesoderm. But the embryology is best expressed and understood clinically in the form of developmental anomalies.

DEVELOPMENTAL ANOMALIES OF THE COLON

Numerous structural developmental anomalies may occur in the colon.

1. **Atresia:**

A. *Membranous atresia*—a complete membrane of varying thickness is stretched across the lumen of the colon, causing complete obstruction.

B. *Saccular atresia*—a segment of the colon ends in a blind pouch with the remainder of the colon present as a tubular structure.

2. **Stenosis:** There is a localized narrowing of the lumen of a segment of bowel, resulting in incomplete obstruction. This may occur in one area or more:

A. *Membranous stenosis*—an incomplete thin diaphragm is stretched across the lumen.

B. *Mural stenosis*—the area of narrowing is thicker than just a membrane, appearing usually as a localized thickening of the wall.

3. **Duplication or triplication,** in which a saccular or tubular structure is attached to the colon and lies between the leaves of the mesocolon. The cavity of the former communicates with the bowel lumen and is lined with contiguous colonic mucous membrane; usually, one wall is common to both the duplication and the colonic segment.

4. **Microcolon**—a uniform reduction in the caliber of a long segment of colon or of the entire colon. The colon is so reduced in caliber as to appear as a miniature colon.

5. **Megacolon**—a uniform dilation of a long segment of colon, usually extending proximally from the rectosigmoid. Congenital megacolon has been ascribed to definite absence of ganglion cells in the myenteric and submucosal (Auerbach's and Meisner's) plexuses in the distal nondilated portion of the bowel wall usually at the rectum and rectosigmoid areas.

Atresia. Localized persistence of the solid stage of the development, that is, failure of one of the epithelial septae to absorb, results in the formation of membranous atresia. If, during the solid stage, epithelial vacuolization so spreads as to cut off a segment (a segment may be pinched off by some unknown reason or mechanism), then a saccular atresia results. Other theories presented to explain atresias include defective intestinal rotation, healed intussusception, vascular anomalies, fetal peritonitis, congenital volvulus and syphilis.

Stenosis. In stenosis there is only partial occlusion of the bowel lumen by a membrane or a thickened wall. It results from persistence of the periphery of the epithelial septae following incomplete recanalization of the solid stage.

Atresias and marked stenoses produce early signs of obstruction in the newborn. They are surgical emergencies that warrant immediate surgical intervention as soon as the diagnosis is made. If left untreated, they are fatal within 1 to 2 weeks. Both atresias and stenoses may be located in more than one segment of the bowel and therefore militate against exploration of the entire bowel, small and large, unless the condition of the patient is in a precarious state. The surgical procedure of choice is primary resection of the involved parts and side-to-side anastomosis for technical facility if the condition of the patient permits. More recently, Gross favors treating colonic atresias by a Mikulicz type of exteriorization of the two blind ends, thus permitting a rapid and aseptic decompression of the proximal bowel. These operations have been attended by very high mortality rates.

Duplications and triplications are rarer than atresias. They are also thought to result from persistence of diverticula which develop normally in some animals and normally should disappear. Or they may result from an isolated coalescence of some vacuoles during the recanalization stage of the solid gastrointestinal tube. These conditions need not necessarily be corrected unless there is an associated pathology at their lower ends where an imperforate anus or fistula may be present, in which case, the latter conditions are treated accordingly.

Microcolon results probably from some extensive defect of the recanalization stage, together with attenuated growth of the involved segment. In half of the reported cases stenosis is associated, and the attention of the surgeon is aroused when signs and symptoms of obstruction occur.

Congenital megacolon (Hirschsprung's disease) has not been understood until about the last 10 years, when its pathogenesis has been attributed to absence of the ganglion cells in Auerbach's and Meisner's plexuses in the myenteric and submucosal plexuses, respectively. The segment involved may measure from 5 to 6 cm. to 20 to 30 cm. in 90 per cent of cases, and these are amenable to surgical correction with very good prognosis. If there is question as to diagnosis, a rectal biopsy of the muscular and submucosal layers should be done preoperatively. Failures in cure after operation have been ascribed to incomplete excision of the involved aganglionic segment of bowel so that frozen sections of the proximal end of the resected bowel may be performed to determine the extent of the diseased segment. In the very young, a transverse colostomy is performed as an initial procedure, followed by a definitive procedure which consists of a sphincter-preserving abdominoperineal resection of the achalasic segment with anastomosis of normally innervated proximal bowel to the extreme terminal rectum or proximal anal canal.

Developmental anomalies also occur in connection with the different stages of rotation.

Derangements of the first stage. These may result in the extroversion of the cloaca with exomphalos. In extroversion of the cloaca, which is seen only in stillbirths, there is an early rupture or an inadequate development of the cloacal membrane, so that the midgut is not extruded. The midgut is seen hanging by a primitive dorsal mesentery and opens near the umbilical region, while lower down both the hindgut and the cloaca open in the anterior abdominal region with the ureteric orifices quite distinct. Failure of the physiologic herniation to reduce results in exomphalos. The small intestine and the right hemicolon may be extruded into the umbilical cord and covered with a fine transparent membrane.

Derangements of the Second Stage. These include nonrotation, reverse rotation and malrotation of the midgut loop. In *nonrotation* of the midgut, the prearterial segment fails to pass to the left side caudal to the artery, with the result that the entire midgut remains suspended by a narrow dorsal attachment, and the colon is nonfixed. The small intestines remain right-sided, the colon left-sided, and the ileum enters the cecum on its right side (instead of as normally on the left side). This may cause volvulus in the newborn, owing to the stimulus of peristalsis following feeding.

In *reverse rotation* the postarterial segment enters the abdomen first and passes to the left behind the artery. The transverse colon lies behind the duodenum and between the superior mesenteric artery and the aorta. The disposition of the small bowel loops otherwise is normal.

Derangement in malrotation may be only partial rotation or combination of both reversed rotation and nonrotation. Usually, internal herniation about the duodenojejunal junction, in any of the numerous fossae, is associated.

Derangements of the Third Stage. These include nonfixation and displacement of viscera, usually with excessive mobility. Imperfect or incomplete descent of the cecum results in subhepatic or lumbar location of the cecum. Excessive descent of the cecum with deficient fixation results in a persistent mesocecum. Deficient fixation of the postarterial mesentery results in a mobile proximal colon with a definite ascending mesocolon. These factors combine to give rise to the mobile cecum. This condition may give rise to intractable, intermittent, right-sided abdominal pain due to intermittent twisting or angulation. When such condition is found on exploration, the mobile cecum is tacked to the posterior abdominal wall with suitably placed silk sutures; or, if its posterior attachment is very little, the latter is incised, and the cecum is allowed to be displaced to the left side of the abdominal cavity (Ladd). The primitive descending mesocolon may persist if there is improper fixation to the posterior abdominal wall.

These derangements of rotation of the bowel should be borne in mind when making a diagnosis of abdominal conditions, as well as on the operating table. Unfamiliarity with these anomalies may cause one to be utterly confused and helpless and waste precious moments figuring out a seemingly complicated problem, thereby placing the patient's life in a very precarious condition. A majority of these cases come to the attention of the surgeon early in neonatal life because of obstructive signs and symptoms. The incompletely rotated cecum may press on the duodenum by virtue of its anterior location and peritoneal attachment on the right posterolateral abdominal wall. This may be associated in about half of the cases with volvulus of the small intestine. When in doubt and when the condition of

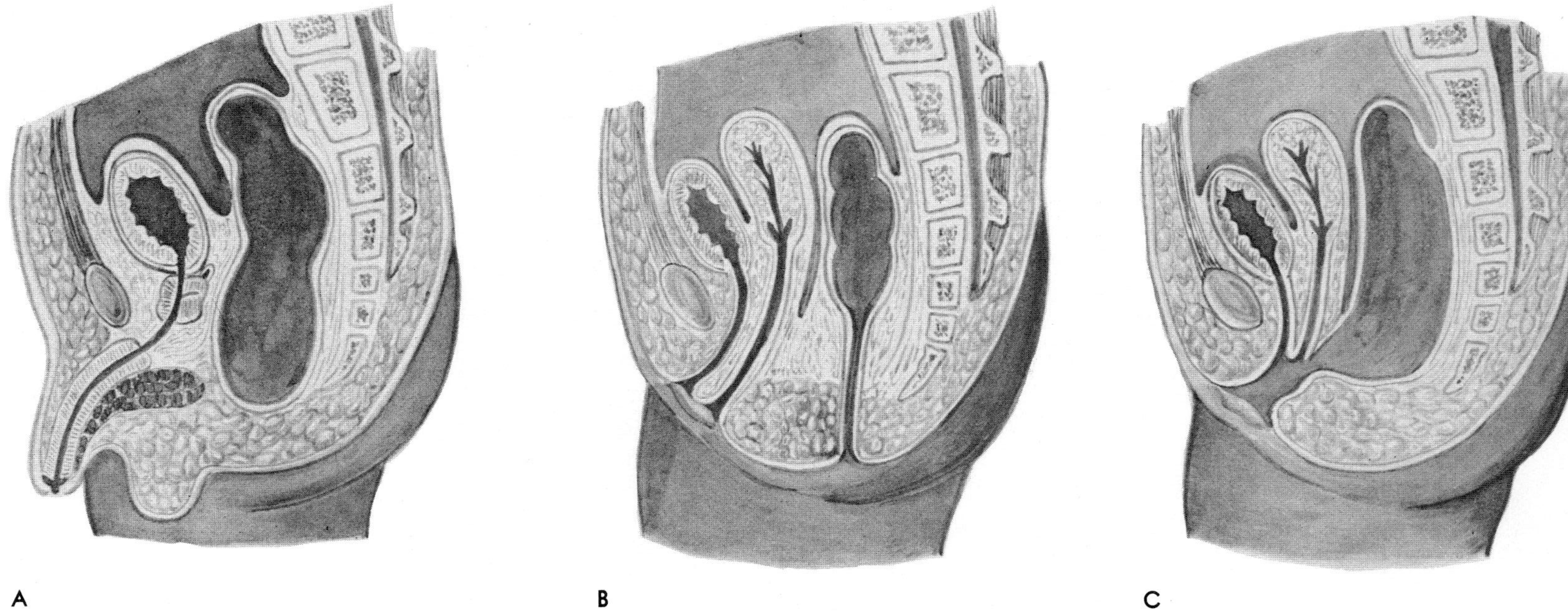

FIG. 8. Anomalies in the development of the pelvic viscera. (A) Failure of the rectum to connect with the anal depression. (B) The anorectal tract is impervious and fibrous. (C) Abnormal anterior location of the anus.

the patient permits, it is advisable to deliver the entire bowel through an adequate wound. The finding on exploration of a generalized bluish discoloration of the small intestine should alert one to the presence of volvulus of the midgut, the twist occurring at the root of the mensentery where a loop or more of small intestine may be found wound around its base. Reduction of the volvulus is carried out by untwisting the mesentery counterclockwise and the change in color of the bowel observed. If cecal malrotation also is noted, the peritoneal band which attaches it to the right posterolateral abdominal wall is incised until the entire duodenum is brought into view and the cecum is allowed to be displaced on the left side of the abdominal cavity.

DEVELOPMENTAL ANOMALIES OF THE RECTUM

Developmental anomalies of the rectum may be either nonfistulous or fistulous.

1. **Nonfistulous Anomalies.** There is no connection between the rectum and the perineum:

A. *Absence of Ampulla.* The rectal ampulla is absent, and the rectal pouch is not so high from the perineum. This could often be brought down by a perineal operation which essentially consists of identifying the blind rectal pouch and bringing it out through the anal sphincters and anchoring it to the perineal skin edges.

B. *Absence of Supra-ampullary Segment.* Both the rectal ampulla and the narrower supra-ampullary segment did not differentiate and are therefore absent. The rectal pouch is rather high. Surgical correction may require a 2-stage procedure: (1) a preliminary transversostomy of the Wangensteen type, followed by (2) a definitive procedure which consists of mobilization of the descending colon and the sigmoid colon and its transplantation to the anal site as a perineal phase.

Persistence of the solid stage of the supra-ampullary segment and/or the ampulla alone results in nonfistulous anomalies of the rectum. A few workers believe that these nonfistulous anomalies may also result from a resorptive process that includes these rectal segments, as occurs usually in the tail gut of the ostrich embryo.

2. **Fistulous Anomalies:**

A. *Rectovesical Fistula or Anovesical Atresia.* The rectum connects with the urinary bladder, usually at the trigone.

B. *Rectourethral Fistula or Anourethral Atresia.* The rectum communicates with the urethra, usually at its membranous portion. It may also open into the prostatic portion and rarely in the penile portion.

C. *Rectovaginal Fistula or Anovaginal Atresia.* The rectum communicates anywhere along the posterior vaginal wall from the level of the cornix to the labia, although it occurs more commonly in the lower third of the vaginal canal.

D. *Rectouterine Fistula or Anouterine Atresia.* The rectum communicates with the uterine cervix or uterine body.

E. *Rectoperineal Fistula or Anoperineal Atresia.* The rectum communicates through an abnormal opening in the perineum. In the male it usually opens at the perineoscrotal junction; in the female the opening usually is caudal to the fourchette.

Fistulous anomalies of the rectum in the male (types A and B, mentioned above) result from failure of the cloacal duct to obliterate. Some workers believe that in these cases the primitive urorectal septum does not even develop, and the

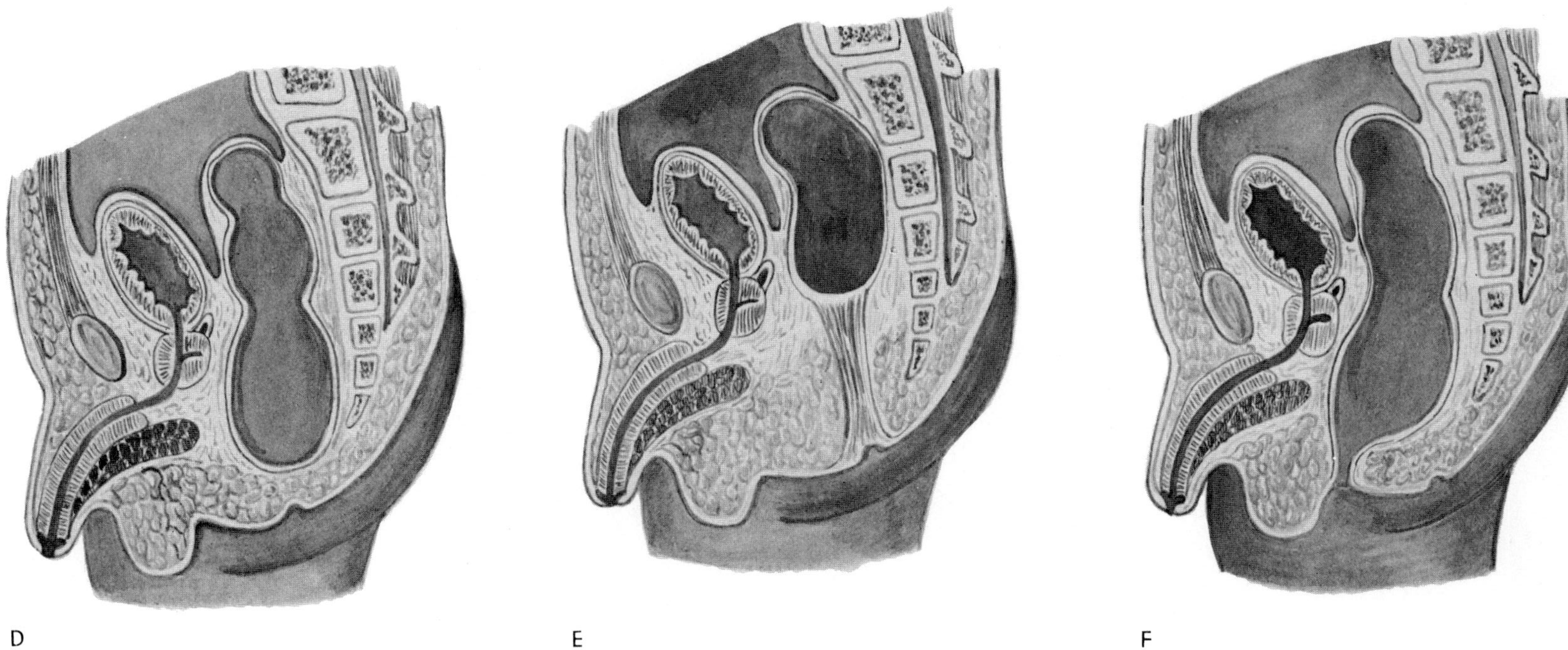

FIG. 9. Anomalies in the development of the pelvic viscera. (D) The lower rectum opens into the vagina; there is complete absence of the anal canal. (E) The rectum opens into the male urethra; part of the anal canal and the terminal rectum are absent. (F) The rectum opens into the bladder; part of the anal canal and the terminal rectum are absent.

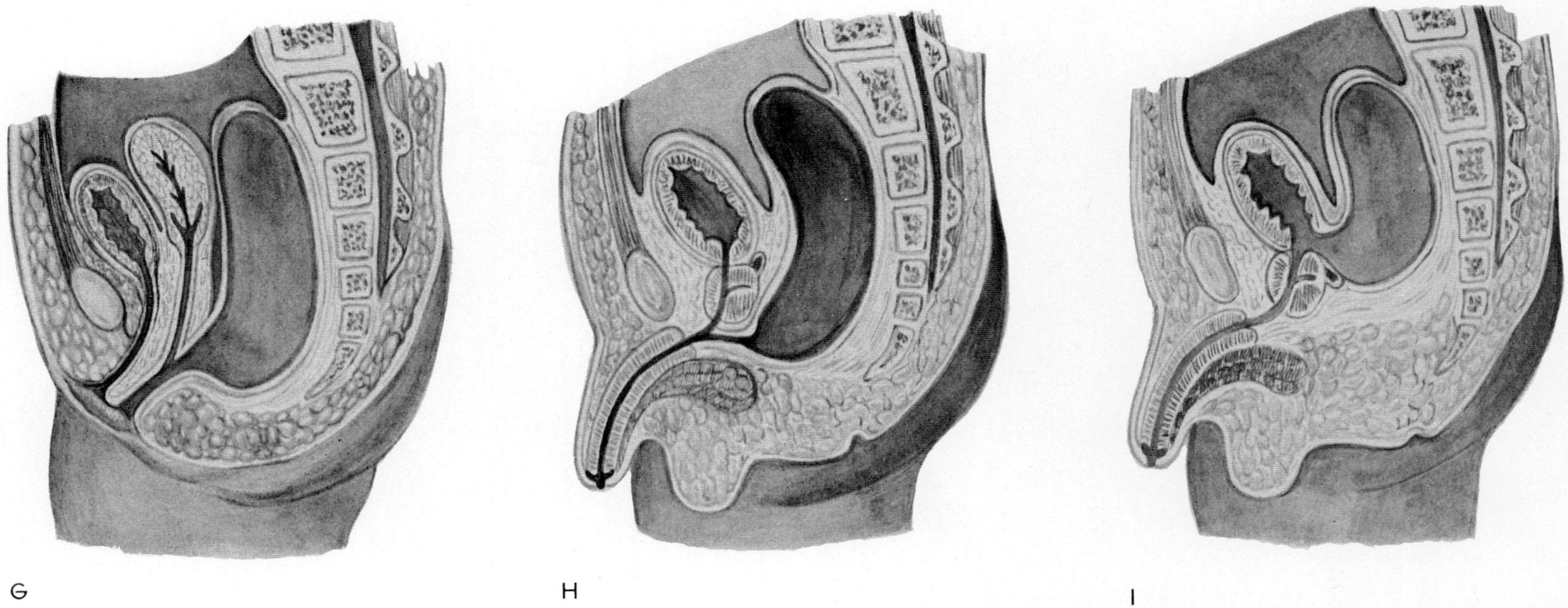

FIG. 10. Anomalies in the development of the pelvic viscera. (G) Complete absence of the anus. (H) The terminal part of the rectum and the anal canal are greatly narrowed. (I) Malformation in which the bladder and the rectum open into a common cavity.

condition could actually be due to persistent primitive cloaca. Fistulous rectal anomalies in the female (types C and D) result from persistent communication between the müllerian ducts and the descending postallantoic gut. Rectouterine fistula results from anomalies of the caudal müllerian ducts. Rectoperineal fistula (type E) results from closure of the anterior portion of the cloacal duct alone, with the posterior portion being carried by the downward growth in this area, with the result that when the cloacal membrane is not involved, the external opening is at the perineum.

Fistulous anomalies involving the rectum and the urinary bladder or the higher portions of the urethra require a preliminary decompression procedure such as a transverse colostomy and a cystostomy; the latter is to prevent retrograde infection. A similar preliminary procedure is required for rectouterine fistula. The definitive procedure consists of excision of the fistulous tract and closure of the openings in the rectum and the urinary bladder or the uterus. Rectovaginal and rectoperineal fistulae are corrected by mobilization of the abnormally placed rectum and transplanting it to the normal anal site.

DEVELOPMENTAL ANOMALIES OF THE ANAL CANAL AND OPENING

There may be occlusion, narrowing, or abnormal location of the anal opening.

1. **Atresia of the Anal Canal.** Occlusion or absence of the anal orifice.

A. *Membranous Occlusion.* There is a complete diaphragm stretched across the anorectal junction, separating the anal canal from the rectum.

B. *Mural Occlusion.* The whole or a segment of the anal canal appears as a solid tube.

2. **Stenosis of the Anal Canal:**

A. *Membranous Stenosis.* An incomplete diaphragm is stretched across the anal canal.

B. *Mural Stenosis.* The site of incomplete obstruction is thicker than a mere membrane and actually involves a short segment of the anal canal.

3. **Abnormal Location of the Anal Opening.** Normally, the anal canal opens in the mid-point of the bi-ischial or interischial plane. When abnormally located, it may open either anterior (more common) or posterior to this point.

Defects in the absorption of the anal or the proctodeal plate are responsible for anomalies of types 1 and 2. In anal anomalies of the membranous type, due consideration must be permitted for the assumption that connective tissue grows into the anal membrane and interferes with its absorption or resorption. In those of the mural type, the connective tissue may be postulated to have grown thickly into the adjacent wall of the rectum, resulting in uniform localized narrowing of the caliber. An improper fusion between the anorectal septum and the cloacal membrane would result in malposition of the opening of the developing anal canal. The commoner anterior malposition is associated with a poorly developed perineal body.

Membranous atresias and stenoses are incised vertically and horizontally, followed by dilatation. Mural atresias require mobilization of the anus until the rectum is reached, which is subsequently brought down. Mural stenosis may respond to simple dilatation or some type of anoplasty, whereas an abnormally placed anus is corrected by mobilization and transplantation to the normal site which is usually marked by a dimple in the perineum, a little posterior to the mid-point of the bi-ischial line.

DEVELOPMENTAL ANOMALIES OF THE SACROCOCCYGEAL AREA

The sacrococcygeal area is the site of a few rare anomalies which may be related to the rectum and the anal canal. In the embryo, the hindgut and the developing neural tube are connected through the neurenteric canal. This canal connects externally with the posterior neural pore. Normally, these openings and channels are obliterated. The postanal gut which develops in the tail fold is normally absorbed or resorbed, as its enveloping tail fold. Among the anomalies in this area are:

1. *Persistent embryonal tail,* which may persist as a fingerlike appendage protruding behind the anal opening.
2. *Persistent neural pore,* which may remain open for a variable distance and is seen as a dimple or as a cranially directed sinus lined by normal skin.
3. *Persistent neural pore and neurenteric canal,* which may remain patent as a small rectosacral fistula.
4. *Persistent postanal gut and neurenteric canal,* to which sacral and retrorectal solid tumors are often traced. Cystic accumulations from secretions of the postanal gut may cause formation of presacral or retrorectal cysts. Though they are of rare occurrence, the tumors that are more commonly found in this region are dermoid cyst, teratoma and chordoma. Dermoids and teratomas may have their origin behind the rectum, in the wall of the rectum or in the rectovaginal septum. A review of the recorded cases shows tumors that arise from the rectal wall to be pedunculated, the base of the pedicle being located approximately 2½ inches above the anus and more frequently on the posterior aspect than anterior. A most unusual case of teratoma having its origin in the sigmoid flexure has been recorded. Surgical extirpation followed by radiotherapy has been the most satisfactory method of treatment for these tumors. The lesion is approached through a mid-line incision extending from the sacrum almost to the anus, and in some cases it may be necessary to sacrifice the coccyx and a small portion of the lowermost segment of the sacrum to obtain exposure. Complete eradication of a chordoma usually is impossible because of its local invasive character, and invariably surgical removal has been attended by recurrence. Radiotherapy has not been very effective.

Chapter 2

Anatomy of Colon, Rectum and Anal Canal

COLON

The colon is a fat-fringed, sacculated tube that is relatively fixed and borders the abdominal and the pelvic cavities. Roughly, it forms a four-sided frame for the disorderly coils of small bowel. Both ends are guarded by circular involuntary sphincters, and there is an apparent progressive decrease in the caliber as one proceeds distally. The decrease in caliber is directly proportional to the increasing thickness of the circular muscle coat and is inversely proportional to the muscular type of the bowel wall, although the large bowel can adapt itself very easily to progressive distention.

The physical habitus and the nutritional state of the individual are reflected

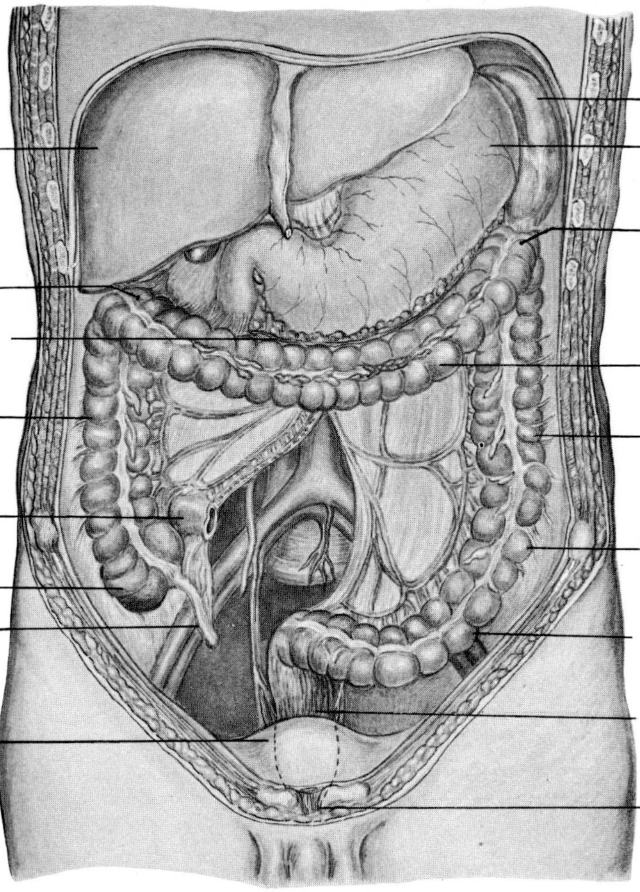

FIG. 11. The relations between the large bowel and the internal organs (front view) with the small bowel and the mesentery removed.

in the physical characteristics of the colon and the mesocolon. Fat, short, stocky individuals have a shorter colon with fatter and less mobile mesocolon in contrast with freely mobile, longer colon of the thin, tall individual.

Certain morphologic characteristics differentiate the large from the small bowel.

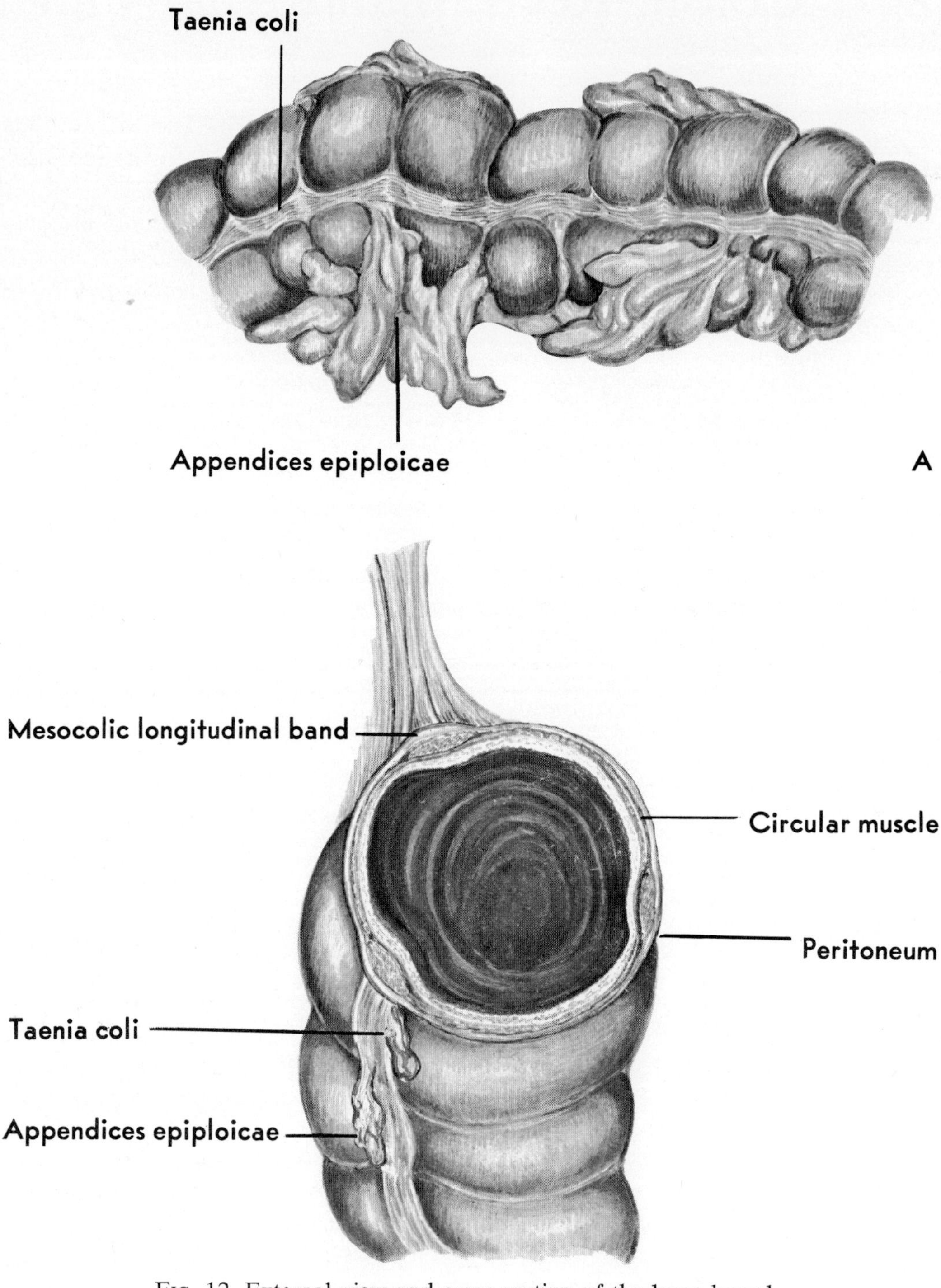

FIG. 12. External view and cross section of the large bowel.

B

1. The large bowel is larger but shorter than the small bowel. The large bowel is only one fourth as long as the small bowel, yet at its narrowest portion, the rectosigmoid, it is still as big as the small bowel. The large bowel decreases in gradual progression from a diameter of 6 to 7.5 cm. (2½ to 3 in.) at the cecum to 2.5 cm. (1 in.) at the rectosigmoid. Owing to its greater distensibility, the colon is called the large bowel, in contradistinction to the small bowel. The relation between large and small bowels as to the length and the diameter depends upon the eating habits of the animal. Herbivorous animals have a long colon and a large cecum suitable for bacterial digestion, while carnivorous animals have a much shorter colon and even a rudimentary cecum which is adaptable for the action of digestive juice. Man, being omnivorous, occupies a position between the two.

2. The colon is more fixed than the jejuno-ileum. Both large and small bowels are attached by the dorsal mesentery to the dorsal body wall during fetal life. But the mesentery proper, which is derived from the mesentery of the midgut, does not undergo absorption or obliteration during its development, so that while the small bowel hangs relatively free from the mesenteric root, it is not fused to the posterior body wall in any of its segments. The small bowel loops are disposed from the left upper quadrant to the right lower quadrant, owing to the oblique line of attachment of the prearterial mesentery.

3. The colon shows taenia coli or linea coli, which start to develop at the age of 3 years. The bowel is generally considered as having 2 distinct layers of smooth muscle: an inner circular and an outer longitudinal layer. It seems that both layers are composed of longitudinal fibers disposed in a spiral manner with varying degrees of obliquity. From the cecum to the rectosigmoid, the longitudinal muscle is bunched into three distinct, equidistant, and equally divided narrow bands ½ cm. wide, called the taenia coli. Over the vermiform appendix the longitudinal muscle forms a complete layer; in fact, its base marks the divergence of the 3 bands. However, some studies have shown the presence of a thin layer of longitudinal muscle fibers between the taenia coli, and thus there would be a complete longitudinal muscle layer in addition to the 3 longitudinal muscle bands. These longitudinal muscle bands are located midanterior, posteromedial and posterolateral in the ascending and the descending limbs. The midanterior band of the vertical limb is not squarely anterior, because during the agglutination of the parietal and visceral layers of the peritoneum there is a contraction of the fibromuscular tissue between them. In the transverse colon there is a shift in the position of the three different taenia, owing to the twisting of the colon during the return of the primitive midgut. Thus, in the final form the midanterior becomes posteroinferior, the posterolateral becomes anterior, and the posteromedial becomes superior in position in the transverse colon. These longitudinal muscle bands converge at the base of the appendix where they form a ring. In relation to the mesocolon these bands are disposed opposite to and equidistant from each side of the mesocolic attachment.

4. The colon, except the cecum, usually has a sacculated appearance unlike the uniform tubulation of the small intestine. Owing to the disproportionate increase in length between the colon and its longitudinal muscle bands, from the 3rd year of life, the colon is bunched up, forming its characteristic saccular haustrations

to adapt 6 feet of colon to only 4 feet of longitudinal muscle bands. Localized condensations of the circular muscles in the colon also helps in the formation of sacculations. Internally, these sacculations or haustral pouches form semilunar folds which encroach upon the lumen of the bowel. The contraction of the bowel in inflammatory processes, as ulcerative colitis, is responsible for the loss of haustrations and the conversion of the gut into a rigid tube. Section of the longitudinal band at the level of a haustration will cause the obliteration of the haustration and result in the lengthening of the bowel segment.

5. The colon presents fat-laden outpouchings of its peritoneal coat called appendices epiploicae. No comparable structure is present in the small bowel. They appear as early as the 5th month of fetal life. These epiploic appendages may occur in one or two rows, and in the vertical limbs they may be related to the anterior and the posteromedial taenia. They are rudimentary and may even be absent altogether, although they are usually discernible over the cecum, the vermiform appendix and the rectum. They are very prominent in the transverse and the sigmoid portions of the colon. In the proximal colon these appendages are flat but tend to be elongated and pedunculated over the sigmoid colon. In the sigmoid colon they appear bifurcate or even trifurcate. These fat tabs are related to the terminal blood vessels of the colon and also serve to surround and hide colonic diverticula. They serve to protect and cushion the terminal vessels when the latter become relatively lengthened as the colon is emptied. They also serve to limit infection within the associated diverticula. The artery inside the epiploic appendage is shorter than its accompanying vein, which pursues a tortuous course about the former. During digestion, the greater weight of the appendices epiploica may predispose to twisting about its pedicle, resulting in necrosis with subsequent calcification and eventual sloughing off, becoming a small yellowish nodule found loose and free in the peritoneal cavity. Such loose bodies are often encountered during the course of a laparotomy. These fat tabs may be used to re-enforce suture lines, especially over an anastomosis.

6. The colon appears white or bluish white, unlike the small bowel, which appears darker owing to congestion that is due probably to the greater vascularity of its walls.

7. Internally, the colon presents a relatively smooth surface except for the semilunar folds of the haustral pouches. It does not possess the circular valvulae conniventes of the small bowel. Neither does it show villi or aggregate lymph nodules. The entire fetal gut has villi, which at the age of 5 to 8 months disappear from the surface of the colon and the rectum.

CECO-APPENDICEAL REGION

The ceco-appendiceal bud develops just beyond the site of the vittelino-intestinal duct at the age of 4 to 5 weeks. Thus embryologically the vermiform appendix is a part of the colon, although it is generally omitted from the surgical problems of the proctologist.

Valves and Sphincters

Generally, the cecum appears as a blind saccular pouch lying in the right iliac fossa at the head of the colon (hence the name caput coli) from the medial wall of which

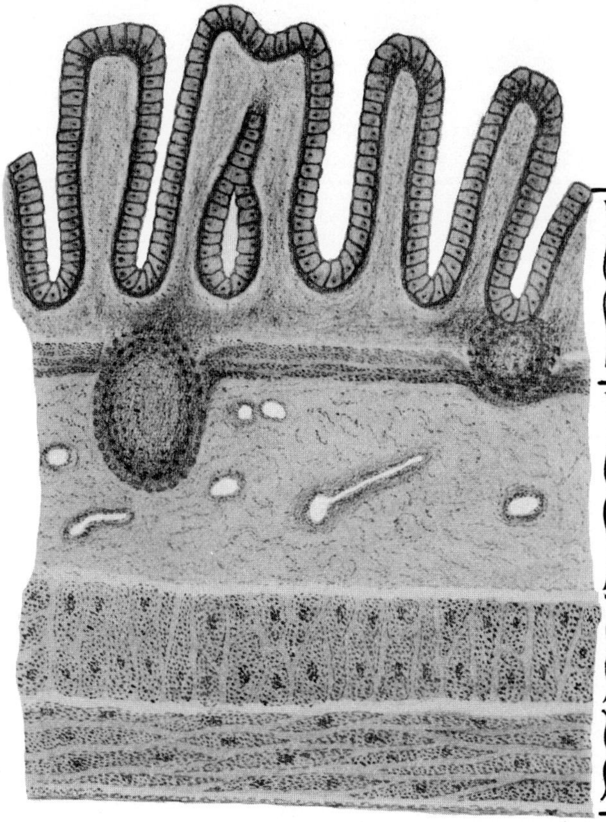

FIG. 13. Microscopic picture of the large bowel (tangentially cut section).

the vermiform appendix arises. The cecum is found below a transverse line passing the ileocecal valve. Into its cavity open the ileum, the appendix and the colon. In fetal life the ileum is thrust at an angle to the cecum, furnishing representation of all the layers. However, the serous coat is replaced by areolar tissue when the 2 layers are in contact. Thus, the ileocecal or ileocolic valve (valve of Bauhinus, Tulpius, Varolius), essentially is composed of the circular muscle of the terminal ileum. The upper lip is derived from the ileum and the ascending colon, but the lower lip from the ileum and the cecum. At this region the circular muscle invaginates into the upper and the lower segments of the ileocecal valve, affording one of the reasons why intussusception so frequently takes place at this site. The ileocecal valve seems to prevent the mixing of the ileal and the colonic contents. Because there is no actual sphincter action, the valve is often incompetent; therefore, diastatic perforations of the cecum and closed loop obstruction do not occur as commonly as expected. If there is a competent ileocecal valve, and closed loop obstruction occurs, the valve will be strong enough to prevent attempts to decompress the obstruction by intubation.

The ceco-appendiceal region is guarded by Guerlach's valve, unless the appendix arises obliquely.

The external boundary between the cecum and the colon is marked by a fur-

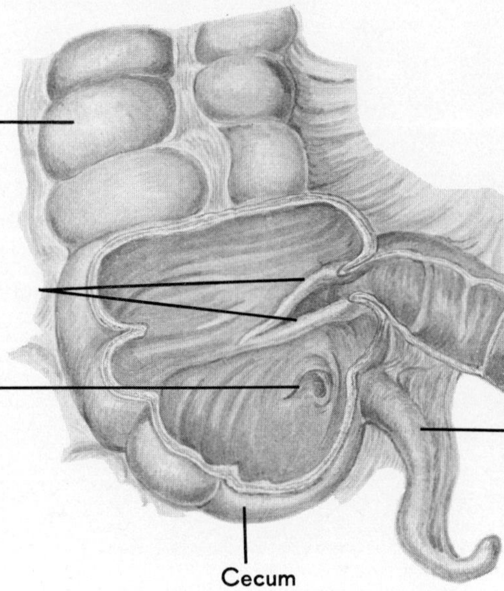

FIG. 14. Interior of ileocecal area.

row that passes partly around the gut and is more marked posteriorly. This marks the site of the first haustration of the colon and has been described as the site of the first sphincter of the colon, the cecocolic sphincter of Busi.

POSITION

The cecum generally is in the right iliac fossa where it lies upon the iliacus and the psoas muscles, the femoral nerve and even the external iliac vessels. Its position varies, depending on the progress of development and fixation of the midgut. It may be located anywhere from a situation near the liver (subhepatic cecum), over the right kidney (lumbar cecum) or low in the pelvis (pelvic cecum). In infants, children and pregnant women, it is found higher than the iliac fossa and gradually descends with advancing age, until in the adult it rests upon the pelvis in the erect position. Its position varies also with the body type of the individual. It is located high in the hypersthenic individual and low in the hyposthenic or asthenic individual. Developmental errors, as malrotation and nonrotation of the midgut loop, are responsible for the location of the cecum in the left side of the abdomen. Despite natural fixation to the body wall, the cecum has been found in sliding hernias, having slid downward and laterally, dragging its peritoneal attachment and investment.

SHAPE

The shape of the cecum varies with its degree of development. Originally, the ceco-appendiceal region has the same diameter as the rest of the colon from which it is derived as an evagination. Later, the lower segment lags in development, and the tapering lower end becomes transformed into the vermiform appendix. The upper half, which develops with the enlarging colon, becomes the cecum. Then the right half develops faster than the left

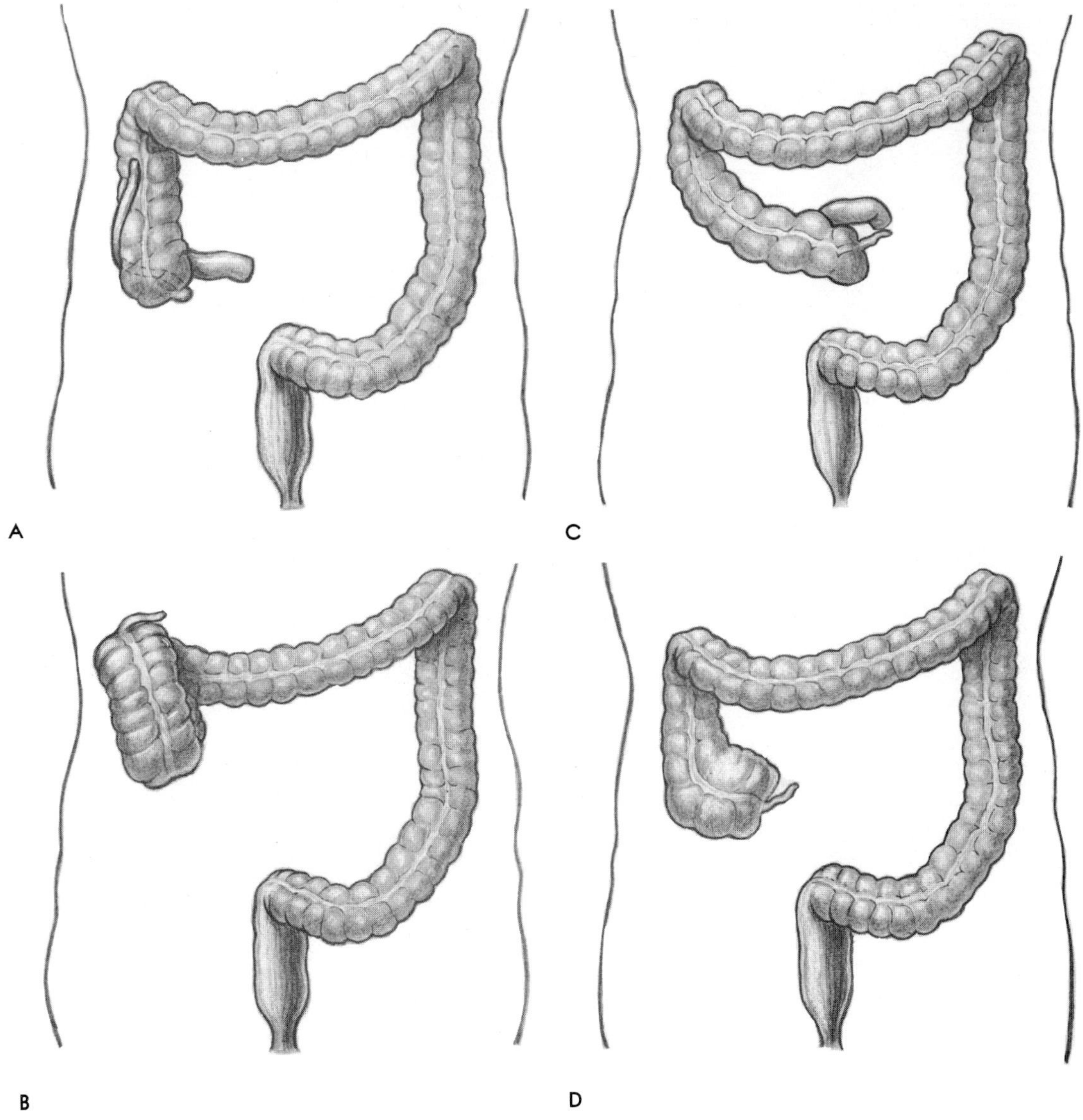

FIG. 15. Variations in the location of the cecum and the appendix.

half, resulting in the asymmetrical cecum. Treves has classified the forms of the cecum as follows:

1. Infantile, 2 per cent incidence: conical cecum merging imperceptibly with the appendix at its apex, as in Hylobates.

2. Quadrate, 3 per cent incidence: the appendix found between the cecum and the longitudinal band.

3. Normal adult type, 90 per cent incidence: the right sacculate larger than the left, a new apex formed, and the appendix directed medially toward the ileocolic junction.

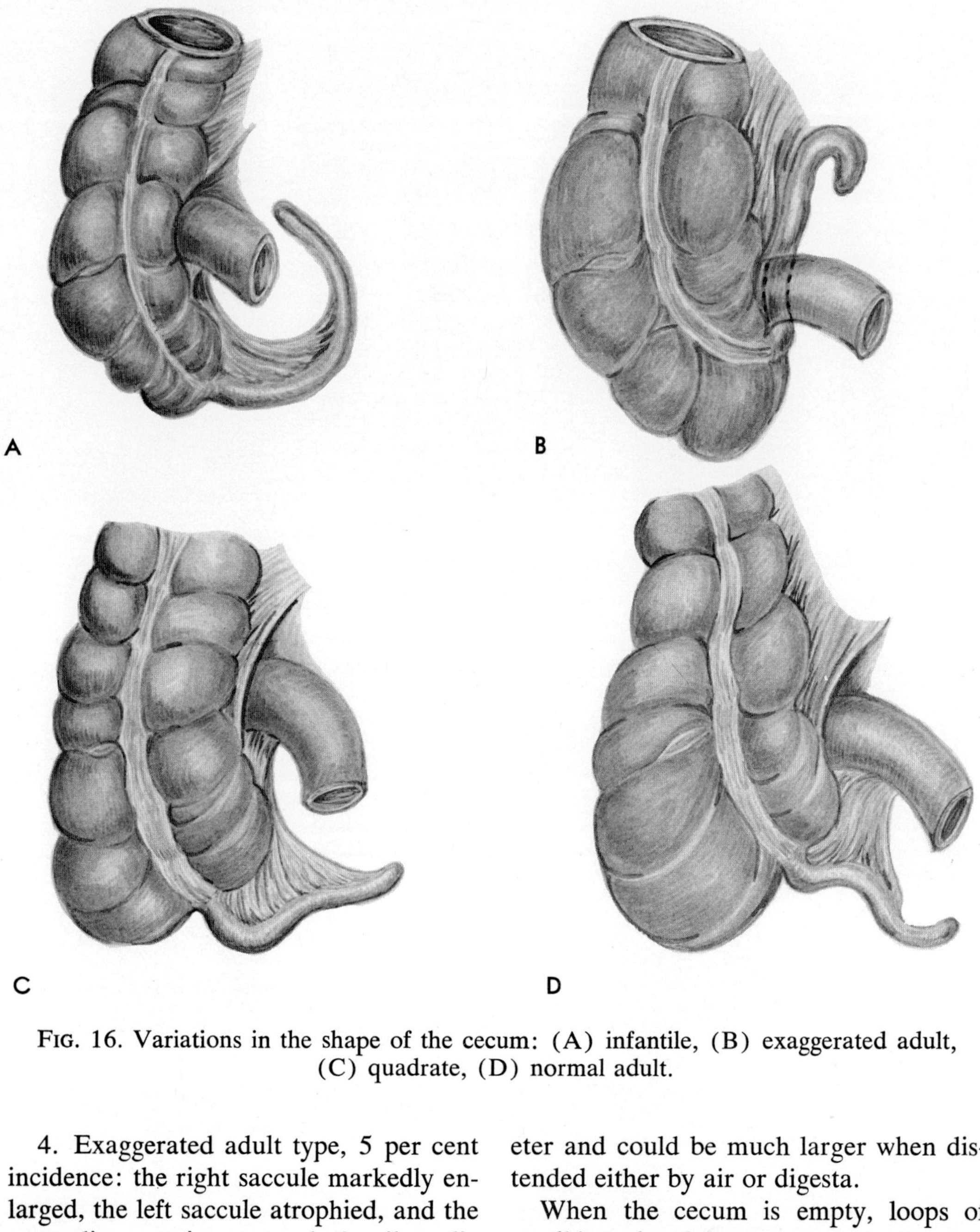

FIG. 16. Variations in the shape of the cecum: (A) infantile, (B) exaggerated adult, (C) quadrate, (D) normal adult.

4. Exaggerated adult type, 5 per cent incidence: the right saccule markedly enlarged, the left saccule atrophied, and the appendix coursing toward the ileocolic junction.

SIZE

The cecum is the largest, thinnest and most superficial part of the colon. Usually it is 6 to 7.5 cm. (2½ to 3½ in.) in diameter and could be much larger when distended either by air or digesta.

When the cecum is empty, loops of small bowel and the greater omentum may be interposed between it and the anterior abdominal wall. The distended cecum touches the abdominal wall and may push away the small bowel and the omentum.

In obstruction of the large bowel distal to the cecum, the latter may rupture

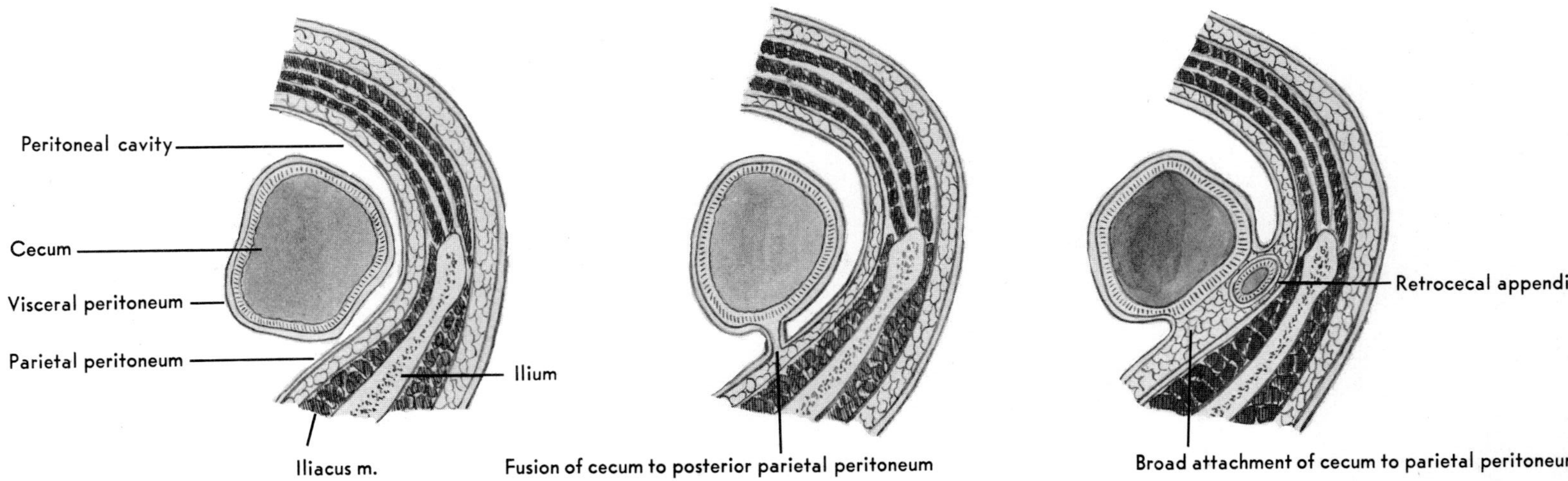

FIG. 17. Cross section at the level of the cecum and the right iliac fossa to show variations in the degree of fusion of the cecum to the parietal peritoneum. (Redrawn)

because its wall is thin and distends easily. In the presence of a competent ileocecal valve, the more proximal the obstruction, the less chance is there for the cecum to hypertrophy, and the greater is the propensity for it to rupture. When the cecum distends, the lips of the ileocecal valve are approximated and closed, but despite them, diastatic perforation is unusual because the ileocecal valve usually is incompetent. During cecal distention there is a prominent out-curving of the flanks, and needle cecostomy in this manner has been performed. In some instances fulness of the cecum may be detected below the costal arches.

Peritoneal Investment

The cecum is covered by peritoneum save for a small area posteriorly where it rests upon the iliacus and the psoas muscles. From the anterior wall, the peritoneum continues onto the ascending colon, but posteriorly the peritoneum is reflected backward and downward over the iliacus muscle, forming the retrocecal recess. When this recess is well developed, it may conceal the vermiform appendix. Normally, the cecum hardly has its own mesentery, although a distinct mesocecum may be noted in 3 out of 20 bodies (15%) examined. A rudimentary fold sufficient to swing the cecum from side to side is present in 2 out of 20 bodies (10%). The cecum may even be fused with the posterior body wall, and its posterior surface may be bare of peritoneum; this occurs in 1 out of 20 bodies (5%). The cecum may be completely invested with peritoneum and be free, with the peritoneum reflected onto the posterior surface of the ascending colon; this occurs in 3 out of every 20 bodies (15%) examined. In some there may be a definite ileocolic mesentery; 1 out of every 20 bodies (5%) examined. Similarly, the cecum and the terminal ileum may be fixed; 1 out of 20 bodies (5%) examined. In a greater number of cases, 4 out of 20 bodies (20%) examined, the peritoneal attachment may be above the ileocecal area. In a few instances, 1 out of 20 bodies (5%), only the terminal ileum is fixed. It may be a distinctly retroperitoneal structure with only its anterior surface covered by peritoneum. When a distinct mesocecum is present, undue mobility of the cecum results, and it may even twist about its mesenteric axis, producing cecal volvulus. It may also descend laterally, forming a right-sided sliding inguinal hernia in which the wall of the sac is the mesocecum folded back. Should its vessels be cut in opening the sac, gangrene of the bowel may supervene. Only the anterior surface will be covered by peritoneum in 2 out of 20 bodies (10%), a condition which is quite common in the apes.

Peritoneal Folds

The cecum and the ascending colon are fixed by numerous accessory peritoneal folds that extend from the posterolateral body wall.

1. *Ileocolic fold (Lockwood, Rolleston),* called also the *superior ileocecal fold of Tuffier and Waldeyer,* the *anterior vascular fold of Moynihan,* the *mesentericocolic fold of Jonnesco.* This fold extends from the anterior surface of the cecocolic area, passes over the ileocolic angle and downward to the root of the appendix. The fold contains the ileocolic artery or the anterior cecal vessels as they pass from the anterior layer of the mesentery of the ileum.

2. *Ileocecal fold (Santorini, von Huschke, Luschka),* called also the *anterior mesoappendix of Clado, intermediary fold of Moynihan,* the *avascular or bloodless fold of Treves.* It extends from the terminal ileum to the mesoappendix or cecum and thus forms a boundary for the superior and the inferior ileocecal fossae.

3. *Mesoappendix,* called also the *mesenteriolum (Bochdalek), posterior vascular fold of Moynihan, inferior ileocecal fold of Waldeyer.* This is the most constant and most important peritoneal fold in this area. It arises from the underlayer of the mesentery proper and serves as the mesentery of the vermiform appendix. It transmits the appendicular vessels. It may not extend beyond the middle of the appendix.

4. *External parietocolic fold,* called also the *right colic ligament of Hensing, cecal ligament of Huschke, superior cecal ligament of Tuffier.* It extends from the posterior surface of the cecum to the posterior body wall and constitutes a peritoneal reduplication the outer portion of which is continuous with the parietal peritoneum extending to the cecum and the ascending colon.

5. *Retrocecal or retrocolic fold (Huschke),* called also the *cecal ligament,* is an avascular fold that extends from the posterior body wall of the iliac fossa across the right paracolic gutter, to the cecum and the ascending colon. It is longer if the peritoneal reflection is higher on the posterior wall of the ascending colon.

6. *Pleurocolic ligament (Langer)* extends from the ascending colon and the cecum to the iliac fascia and may even fuse with the false capsule of the right kidney.

7. *Nephrocolic ligament (Longyear)* is considered by some as being merely the deeper fibers of the external parietocolic fold. It extends from the posterior surface of the cecum and the ascending colon to the false capsule of the right kidney. These fibers usually fuse with those of the nephrocolic ligament and have been considered as only part of the latter.

8. *Intra-angular fold (Engel),* called also *mesentericoparietal fold of Jonnesco, inferior cecal ligament of Tuffier,* extends from the mesentery of the terminal ileum to the posterior parietal wall and probably represents a remnant of the genitomesenteric fold of Reid. This fold is quite prominent in the fetus.

9. *Internal parietocolic fold* is the medial homolog of the external parietocolic fold and extends from the medial border of the cecal pouch to the posterior body wall.

10. *Ileal membrane (Lane's membrane).* This is an avascular fold of parietal peritoneum extending from the right iliac fossa to the antimesenteric border of the terminal ileum. It was thought to cause kinking or obstruction on contraction. Occasionally, it pulls the terminal ileum to the right side with the vermiform appendix concealed beneath it. Because it is avascular it may be cut with impunity to expose the appendix.

Peritoneal Recesses

Several peritoneal recesses are formed by the different peritoneal folds. The vermiform appendix may become enclosed in any of these pericecal fossae, or an internal hernia may develop.

1. *Ileocolic fossa (Luschka, Lockwood, Rolleston),* called also *superior cecal fossa (Hartman, Treves, Tuffier, Waldeyer), ileocecal recess of Broesike, or anterior*

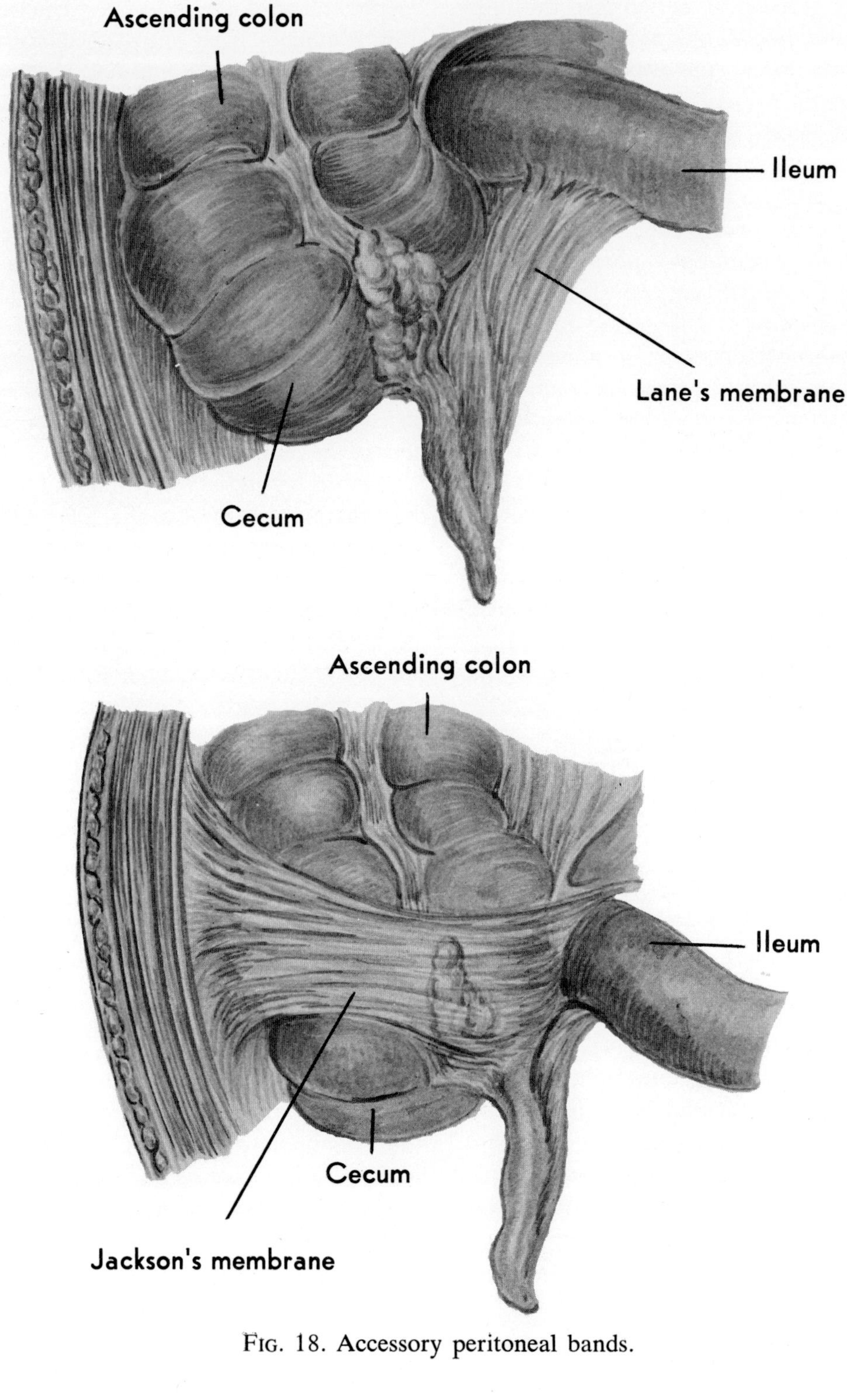

FIG. 18. Accessory peritoneal bands.

ileocolic fossa, bounded posteriorly by the ascending colon, anteriorly by the ileocolic fold, which contains the ileocolic artery and vein. It is above the ileocolic junction, opens to the left and lies on the terminal ileum. It is quite prominent in children and thin individuals.

2. *Ileocecal fossa (Huschke, Lockwood, Rolleston, Kelynack and Berry),* called also inferior ileocecal recess *(Lacuet, Treves, Tuffier, Waldeyer) or ileo-appendicular fossa of Clado and of Moynihan.* It is bounded anteriorly by the ileocecal fold, posteriorly by the meso-appendix, and superiorly by the posterior surface of the ileum. It may be deep enough to extend beneath the ascending colon up to the level of the right kidney and even the duodenum. This fossa should be investigated first in the course of an appendectomy if the appendix is not found in its usual position.

3. *Retrocecal fossa (Jonnesco)* called also *retrocolic fossa (Moynihan, Treves, Berry, Broesike) or subcolic fossa (Lockwood and Rolleston).* It is bounded anteriorly by the posterior surface of the cecum, posteriorly by the iliac fossa; to the right lies the right paracolic gutter, and to the left the mesentery. It may be divided into two by a secondary fold. It is of varying depth, depending upon the height of the level of the peritoneal reflection on the posterior wall of the ascending colon. The appendix frequently is lodged in the so-called retrocecal position in about 60 per cent of cases.

4. *Retro-appendicular fossa (Hartman, Leichtenstein),* called also *postileac recess of Tarenetzky,* is an inconstant dimple between the intra-angular fold and the mesoappendix.

Supports of the Cecum

The cecum is held in place by: (1) continuity with the terminal ileum and the ascending colon; (2) investing peritoneum which fixes it against the posterior body wall; (3) mesocecum, if present; (4) peritoneal ligaments and folds as enumerated above; (5) normal intra-abdominal pressure.

ASCENDING COLON

Size, Shape and Location

The ascending colon is that segment between the cecocolic furrow and the right colic or hepatic flexure. It varies in length, depending upon the level of the cecum, although generally it is 12.5 to 20 cm. (5 to 8 in.) long. It extends upward along the right side of the abdominal cavity from the cecum to the inferior surface of the right lobe of the liver. In cases with subhepatic cecum the ascending colon may be looped medially. In other instances it may be redundant and elongated. It rarely moves and appears as a short tube, generally only half as long as the descending segment of the colon.

Position and Relations

Anteriorly, it is separated by some coils of jejuno-ileum and the fringe of the greater omentum from the anterior body wall. Posteriorly, it is related from above downward with the perirenal fat and the capsule of the right kidney, the anterior layer of the lumbodorsal fascia on the right, and the iliacus fascia (as they cover the quadratus lumborum and the iliacus muscles, respectively). It may also be related at this point to the aponeurosis of the transversus abdominis muscle. Because the ascending colon overlies the right kidney, percussion over renal tumors may evoke tympanitic sound or note.

The colon may be lacerated in the course of dissection and separation of a

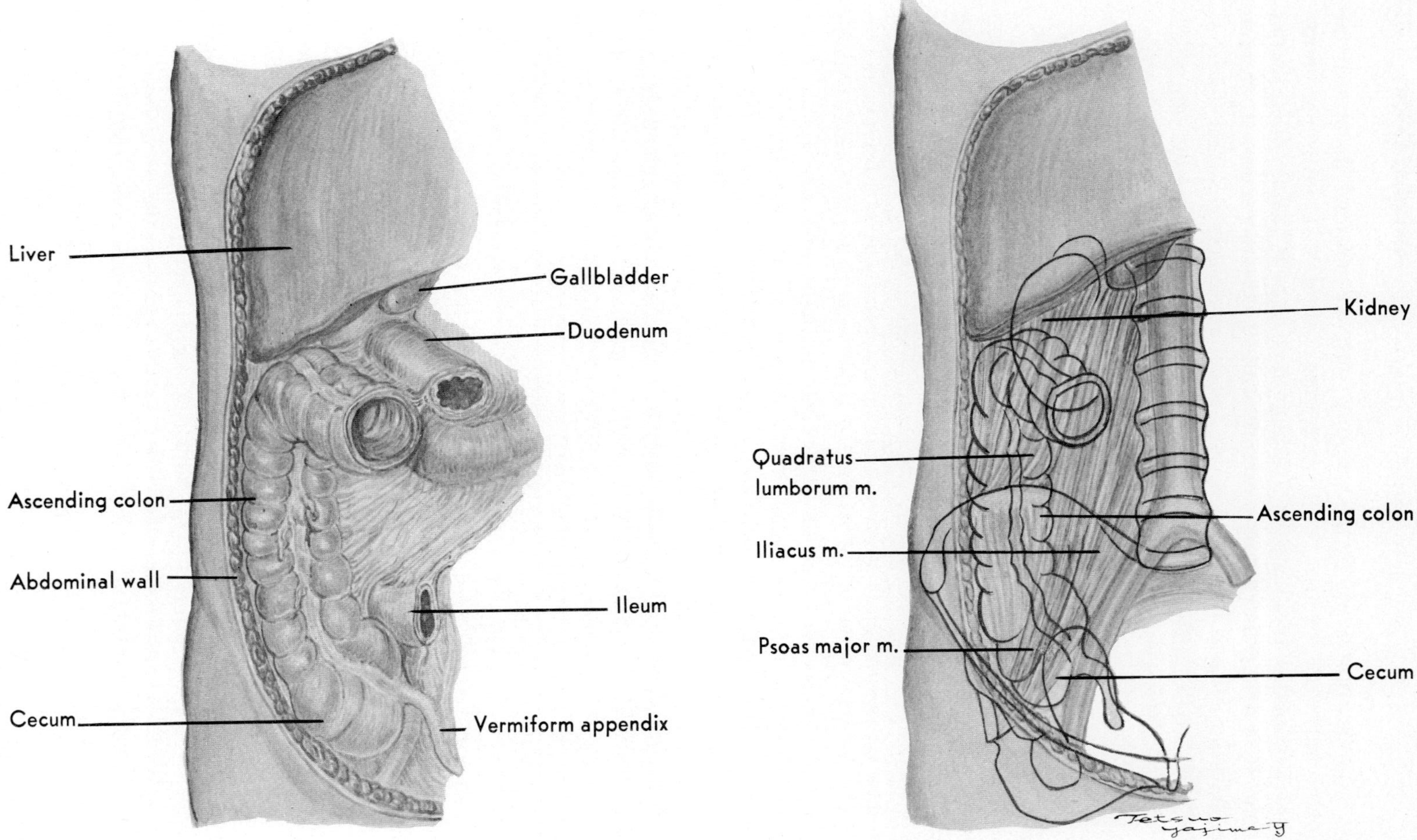

FIG. 19. The ascending colon, its position and relations.

pyonephrotic capsule. Perinephric abscesses may empty into the colon. Between the ascending colon and the lower pole of the right kidney is found Toldt's fusion fascia. This fascia forms an avascular cleavage plane that separates the ascending colon from the kidney. In transperitoneal right-sided nephrectomy, this fascia should be dissected free from the ascending colon. Laterally, it is separated from the body wall by the right paracolic gutter. Medially, the ascending colon is related from above downward with the following structures in the right infra-omental or the medial infracolic compartment—the descending portion of the duodenum, some small bowel coils, and the areolar tissue that covers the psoas major muscle. Medially and posteriorly in the loose areolar tissue are found the ureter and the gonadal (spermatic or ovarian) vessels of the right side.

Peritoneal Investment

The ascending colon is covered by visceral peritoneum anteriorly, medially and laterally in one half of the bodies examined. The peritoneal covering binds this portion to the posterior and the lateral body walls. The lateral peritoneal attachments are along the physiologic line of fusion between the parietal and the visceral peritoneum. The ascending colon should be fixed in order to enable it to support the bowel, propel the fluid fecal column against gravity and prevent fecal stasis. Its posterior wall may be invested by peritoneum to a varying extent, and a definite ascending mesocolon may be demonstrated in 1 out of every 4 bodies examined.

The persistence of the ascending mesocolon results in a mobile ascending colon. This could induce cecal stasis, cecal volvulus and ileocecal intussusception. Arteriomesenteric or duodenal ileus results from compression by the superior mesenteric vascular pedicle over the duodenum against the lumbar vertebrae, if there is cecal stasis which pulls down on the vascular pedicle. A mobile cecum or mobile ascending colon will induce the cecum to twist about itself or about an adjacent coil of small intestine, resulting in cecal volvulus.

Peritoneal Folds

Numerous peritoneal attachments are present between the ascending colon and the body wall and the surrounding viscera. Usually, a few of these peritoneal folds or ligaments are also related to the posterior cecal wall. Among them are: (1) retrocolic fold of Huschke (described previously under cecum); (2) pleurocolic ligament of Langer (described previously under cecum); (3) nephrocolic ligament of Longyear (described previously under cecum).

The peritoneal folds of the ascending colon proper include:

1. *Parietocolic fold of Flint,* that extends from the ascending colon to the parietal wall and is often inserted into the line of physiologic fusion between the visceral and parietal peritoneum.

2. *Pericolic membrane of Jackson*—a membranous peritoneal fold that extends from the posterior abdominal wall downward and inward to the anterior longitudinal band of the ascending colon. Numerous fine straight long vessels run parallel with one another in this membrane. The vessels rarely, if ever, require ligation, and Jackson's membrane usually can be cut with impunity without incurring any serious consequence.

3. *Hepatic ligament,* that extends from the ascending colon to the anterolateral abdominal wall at the level of the iliac

crest. Because the inferior margin of the right lobe has been seen to rest upon it, this ligament has been called the sustentaculum hepatis (homologous with the sustentaculum lienis or the phrenocolic ligament).

4. *Ascending mesocolon,* which results from the persistence of the primitive ascending mesocolon. It may be demonstrated in 1 out of 4 bodies examined.

Fixation and Support

The ascending colon is held in place by: (1) continuity with the cecum below and with the hepatic flexure above; (2) investing peritoneum that fixes it against the posterior body wall; (3) ascending mesocolon, if present; (4) peritoneal ligaments and folds; (5) normal intra-abdominal pressure.

HEPATIC FLEXURE

Position and Relations

From the ascending colon, the contiguous right colic or hepatic flexure turns downward and twists forward, acutely as a rule, between the inferior margin of the right lobe of the liver and the posterior surface of the lower pole of the right kidney. On both organs it causes colic impressions. The hepatic flexure passes downward and forward to join the transverse colon. Anteromedially, it is related to the fundus of the gallbladder. This proximity to the gallbladder enables gallstones to produce erosion through an acutely inflamed gallbladder into the lumen of the colon. Posteromedially lies the descending portion of the duodenum and the right kidney. Usually, its peritoneal investment is complete except posteriorly.

The hepatic bend or right colic angle is almost invariably lower, less acutely flexed, more superficial, and not as well supported as the splenic flexure.

Peritoneal Ligaments

Several ligaments lie at and help to fix

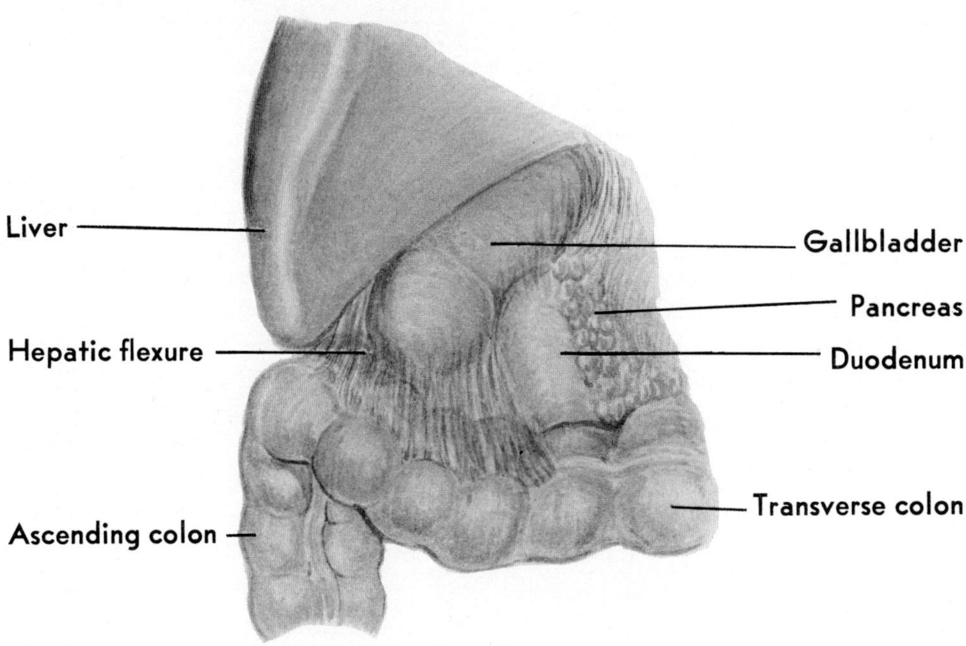

Fig. 20. Hepatic flexure and its relations.

the hepatic flexure. The flexure has some degree of mobility, usually 2.5 cm. (1 in.), although in some individuals it may be as much as 7.5 cm. (3 in.), especially if there is a persistent ascending mesocolon. Among the peritoneal ligaments are:

1. *Hepatocolic or hepatocolonic ligament,* at times referred to as the *hepatoduodenal ligament.* It extends from the lesser omentum or gastroduodenal ligament, passes downward to the right end of the right colic flexure.

2. *Duodenal ligament or cystoduodenal ligament* that extends from the gallbladder across the duodenum to the hepatic flexure and is present in 3 or 4 out of every 10 bodies examined.

3. *Nephrocolic ligament of Longyear* that extends from the posterior surface of the hepatic flexure with fibers from the ascending colon and forms part of the false capsule of the right kidney.

Fixation and Support

The hepatic flexure is held in place by: (1) continuity with the ascending and the transverse portions of the colon; (2) investing peritoneum, fixing it to the posterior body wall; (3) greater omentum which pulls it upward and also presses it against the posterior body wall; (4) peritoneal ligaments and folds, especially the duodenocolic and the cysticocolic ligaments; (5) normal intra-abdominal pressure; and (6) its vascular pedicles.

TRANSVERSE COLON

Position and Length

The transverse colon is the longest and most fixed and most easily identified segment of the colon. It stretches across the abdomen, running slightly upward, from right to left, between the two fixed colic flexures between which it sags. It always possesses a definite transverse mesocolon. The transverse colon measures from 40 to 50 cm. (16 to 20 in.) long and is roughly one third of the length of the entire large bowel. The transverse colon becomes longer if the cecum is undescended, and if the transverse mesocolon is long. As the ascending colon bends to form the right colic flexure, there is a twist so that the anterior surface faces posteriorly, the anterolateral aspect faces superiorly, and the posteromedial aspect faces inferiorly.

In 4 out of 5 individuals, in the erect position, the transverse colon does not sag below the level of the umbilicus. In females, the degree of sagging is a trifle lower, and the segment is consequently longer than in males. Among males, it may sag 7.5 to 10 cm. (3 to 4 in.) below the level of the iliac crests, as compared with 10 to 12.5 cm. (4 to 5 in.) in females. Because the transverse colon lies lower in the female, it is more liable to be involved in pelvic inflammatory disease, and come to adhere to the uterus, the fallopian tubes and the ovaries. Pendulous transverse colons with long mesocolon have been found within umbilical and ventral hernial sacs, and even within femoral and inguinal hernial sacs.

Relations

Because it is the longest and least-fixed segment of the colon, and since it runs across the abdomen, the transverse colon is related to more structures than any other segment of the large bowel. Anteriorly lie the 2 layers of greater omentum, at times separated by coils of small bowel from the anterior body wall. Posteriorly, it is related to the descending portion of the duodenum, the head of the pancreas, the anterior layer of the lumbosacral fascia, and more small bowel coils. Superiorly may be found the liver and the gallbladder on the right end, and the greater curvature of the stomach and the lower end of the spleen on the left end. Inferiorly are found coils of jejuno-ileum. An acutely inflamed gallbladder or a large liver abscess may perforate into the transverse colon, owing to the proximity to the gallbladder and liver respectively. Similarly, a carcinoma of the stomach may by direct extension perforate into the transverse colon and give rise to a gastrocolic fistula.

Peritoneal Investment

The transverse colon is almost entirely invested with peritoneum, except posteriorly where its long transverse mesocolon is a bilaminar structure of varying adiposity, length and mobility. The structure forms a sloping horizontal partition stretched across the upper abdomen attached along the whole length of the posterior surface of the transverse colon. Because of this anatomic fact it is called the secondary diaphragm of Henle. Here the peritoneum is a fan-shaped structure, being wider at its attachment to the colon than at its origin. It originates from the anterior surface of the head, the neck and the body of the pancreas; occasionally, it extends further to the right, crossing the descending portion of the duodenum. At each end, the peritoneum is related to the inferior pole of each kidney; it is wider at the middle than at the flexures which lie deeper. As a result, the transverse colon sags and is more mobile in the middle portion while it is fixed at the flexures. This transverse partition divides the abdominal cavity into a supramesocolic compartment above, and an inframesocolic compartment below. Because the greater omentum adheres to part of the upper half of the transverse mesocolon, the omental bursa (lesser peritoneal sac) is also separated from the inframesocolic compartment.

Greater Omentum

Another structure intimately related to the colon is the greater omentum, whose attachment is the identifying characteristic of the transverse colon. As a structure, it has 4 layers and forms a compound peritoneal fold that develops from the dorsal mesogastrium, which has continued to grow even after the definitive rotation of the stomach. Hence, it is attached along the greater curvature of the stomach, descends into the abdominal cavity, folds upon itself and ascends on the posterior body wall where it fuses with the diaphragm. In the embryo an omental cavity, lined by peritoneum, is thus formed and is found between the 2nd and the 3rd layers. This omental cavity normally is obliterated by fusion of the apposing layers below the level of the transverse colon, although it may persist until adulthood. During intra-uterine life, the posterior or 4th layer of the great omentum fuses with the serosa of the transverse colon, and the transverse mesocolon obliterates the space between itself and the greater omentum, making the transverse mesocolon form part of the floor of the omental bursa. This line of fusion is detectable in the adult and forms an avascular cleavage plane along which the epiploic vessels may be separated from the transverse mesocolon and the transverse colon without troublesome bleeding obscuring the field. The gastrocolic ligament is that part of the greater omentum above the level of the transverse colon that seems to join the greater curvature of the stomach to the transverse colon. The layers of the greater omentum generally are adherent up to the level of the transverse colon, and so the greater omentum seems to arise from the concavity of the transverse colon. Owing to the fusion between the greater omentum and the transverse mesocolon, the middle colic artery which lies in the transverse mesocolon may be ligated accidentally, causing possibly disastrous results while performing a gastrectomy.

PERITONEAL FOLDS AND LIGAMENTS

Numerous peritoneal folds and ligaments pass from the transverse colon to the related structures.

1. *Cystogastrocolic or cystocolic ligament:* extends from the gallbladder across the duodenum to the transverse colon and is closely related to the more laterally placed cysticoduodental ligament.

2. *Gastrocolic ligament:* extends from the greater curvature of the stomach to the transverse colon and represents the anterior unfused part of the greater omentum above the level of the transverse colon.

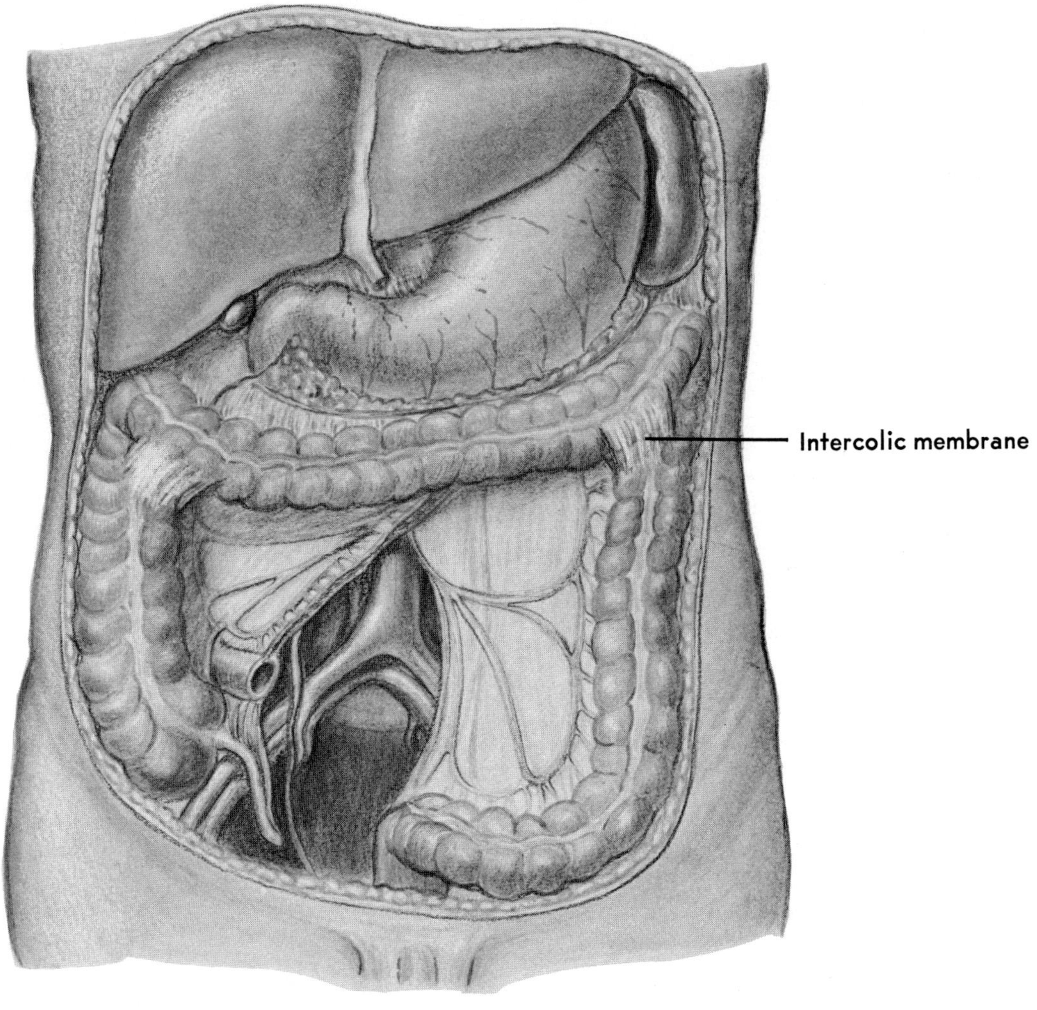

FIG. 21. The intercolic membranes.

3. *Mesocolicojejunal fold or transverse intramesentericocolic fold of Broesike:* extends from the undersurface of the transverse mesocolon to the antimesenteric border of the proximal jejunum and even under the superior mesenteric artery.

4. *Right intercolic membrane:* a membranous connection between the contiguous medial border of the transverse colon and the ascending colon at the hepatic flexure.

5. *Left intercolic membrane of Payr* is the homolog of the right intercolic membrane and is found at the contiguous medial border of the transverse colon at the splenic flexure. These intercolic membranes have been thought to cause an acute reduplication of the colon upon itself, resulting in a double-barreled obstructed colon.

Fixation and Supports

The transverse colon is relatively fixed only at both ends, through the colic flexures. Otherwise, it is held in place by (1) continuity with the vertical limbs of the colon at the flexures or bends; (2) the transverse mesocolon and the peritoneal investment; (3) numerous peritoneal folds and ligaments that join it to the nearby structures; (4) its vascular pedicle; and (5) normal intra-abdominal pressure.

SPLENIC FLEXURE

In its distal aspect, the transverse colon is directed upward, backward and to the left, beneath the ribs where, just below the level of the lower angle of the spleen, it bends acutely downward to form the splenic flexure (left colic flexure), and then continues as the descending colon. The splenic flexure lies higher, is deeper and more acute than the hepatic flexure because the left lobe of the liver is smaller than the right. With the exception of the rectum, the splenic flexure is the most fixed part of the large bowel as well as the most inaccessible. To mobilize the splenic flexure, the paramedian incision should be prolonged to the left costal arch. In slender individuals, a vertical prolongation is enough, but in obese individuals an angular prolongation not unlike a hockey stick may be necessary. Preoperatively, an examination of the roentgenogram of a filling barium enema may be helpful and enough to give one an idea of the height of the splenic flexure under the rib cage.

Relations

The splenic flexure is overlaid by the body of the stomach and part of the left lobe of the liver and lies on the perirenal fat and fascia on the outer border of the left kidney, the left crus of the diaphragm, and the left transversus abdominis muscle. Posteriorly, it it attached to the tail of the pancreas, by the left end of the transverse mesocolon. Above and to the left is the spleen as it lies supported by the sustentaculum lienis or the phrenocolic ligament.

Peritoneal Investment

Usually, its peritoneal investment is complete, leaving only a bare area posteriorly just like the other colonic segments. Then it may well be enclosed completely and be attached posteriorly to the tail of the pancreas by a distinct fold from the left end of the greater omentum, posteriorly by the attachment of the transverse mesocolon and the pancreas. Laterally, it is fixed by the phrenicocolic ligament (costocolic ligament).

Peritoneal Folds and Ligaments

The peritoneal folds and ligaments in relation to the splenic flexure include:

1. *Phrenicocolic or costocolic ligament:* a triangular ligament which extends from the lateral aspect of the flexure and is directed upward and inward to the diaphragm at the region of the 10th and the 11th ribs, although occasionally it may extend up to the 9th rib. Upon its lower portion rests the spleen, and it may be called sustentaculum lienis or the suspensory ligament of the spleen. While it is usually an avascular fold, in diseases affecting the distal transverse or proximal descending colon one or more large engorged vessels usually are present in this ligament which require ligation.

2. *Intercolic membrane of Payr,* mentioned above in connection with the transverse colon.

Fixation and Supports

The splenic flexure is well fixed and is held by: (1) contiguity with the transverse and the descending portions of the colon; (2) its vascular pedicle; (3) peritoneal ligaments, especially the phrenicocolic ligament; and (4) normal intra-abdominal pressure.

DESCENDING COLON

The descending colon extends from the splenic flexure down to the pelvic brim. The iliac colon, or that portion that overlies the iliac bone, is considered by some to be the fixed component of the iliopelvic colon in contradistinction to its more mobile pelvic segment. Because the iliac colon is fixed like the ascending colon, it may be more justifiable to consider this entire fixed segment as the descending colon divided into a lumbar and an iliac segment. The lumbar descending colon has more prominent appendices epiploicae. As the splenic flexure bends downward there is a change in the direction of the taenia coli. The descending colon is more than twice the length of the ascending colon; although it is narrower than the ascending colon, it is usually a foot longer than the latter.

Relations

The descending colon starts more laterally and is more deeply placed than the ascending colon. It descends vertically, inclining medially to curve across the lower pole of the left kidney, where it assumes a more medial position. Then the lumbar portion descends vertically, lying lateral to the left ureter and over the quadratus lumborum fascia as far as the iliac bone as the iliac colon descends down to the pelvic brim. The descending colon turns medially across the left psoas major muscle and ends as the pelvic colon in front of the external iliac artery. Posteriorly, the bowel rests, from above downward, on the inferior surface of the left half of the diaphragm, anterior layer of the left lumbodorsal fascia, left iliac and left psoas fascia, which cover respectively the quadratus lumborum, the iliacus and the psoas muscles. Laterally, the left lateral paracolic gutter separates the descending colon from the body wall, while anteromedially are coils of small bowel as they lie in the left half of the inframesocolic compartment. The greater omentum usually separates the descending colon from the abdominal wall. The lower half crosses several vessels and nerves, the latter lying beneath the respective fascial covering of the different muscles mentioned above, Hence, it crosses the ilioinguinal and the iliohypogastric nerves in the region of the quadratus lumborum; the lateral cutaneous nerve of the thigh and the iliac branch of the iliolumbar artery at the region of the iliacus; and the femoral nerve and the external iliac vessels at the psoas major muscle. The genitofemoral nerve and the gonadal vessels (testicular or ovarian) lie close to the left external iliac artery where the iliac segment passes across the pelvic or the sigmoid colon. Owing to its relation to the left kidney, the lumbar portion of the descending colon may be injured in the course of dissecting left-sided pyonephrosis. Left perinephric abscesses or calculous pyonephrosis may perforate into the large bowel. The ureter and the left gonadal vessels may be adherent to the posterior parietal peritoneum and may be injured in operations on the left colon unless properly separated.

Peritoneal Investment

In 2 out of 3 the descending colon is generally invested with peritoneum ante-

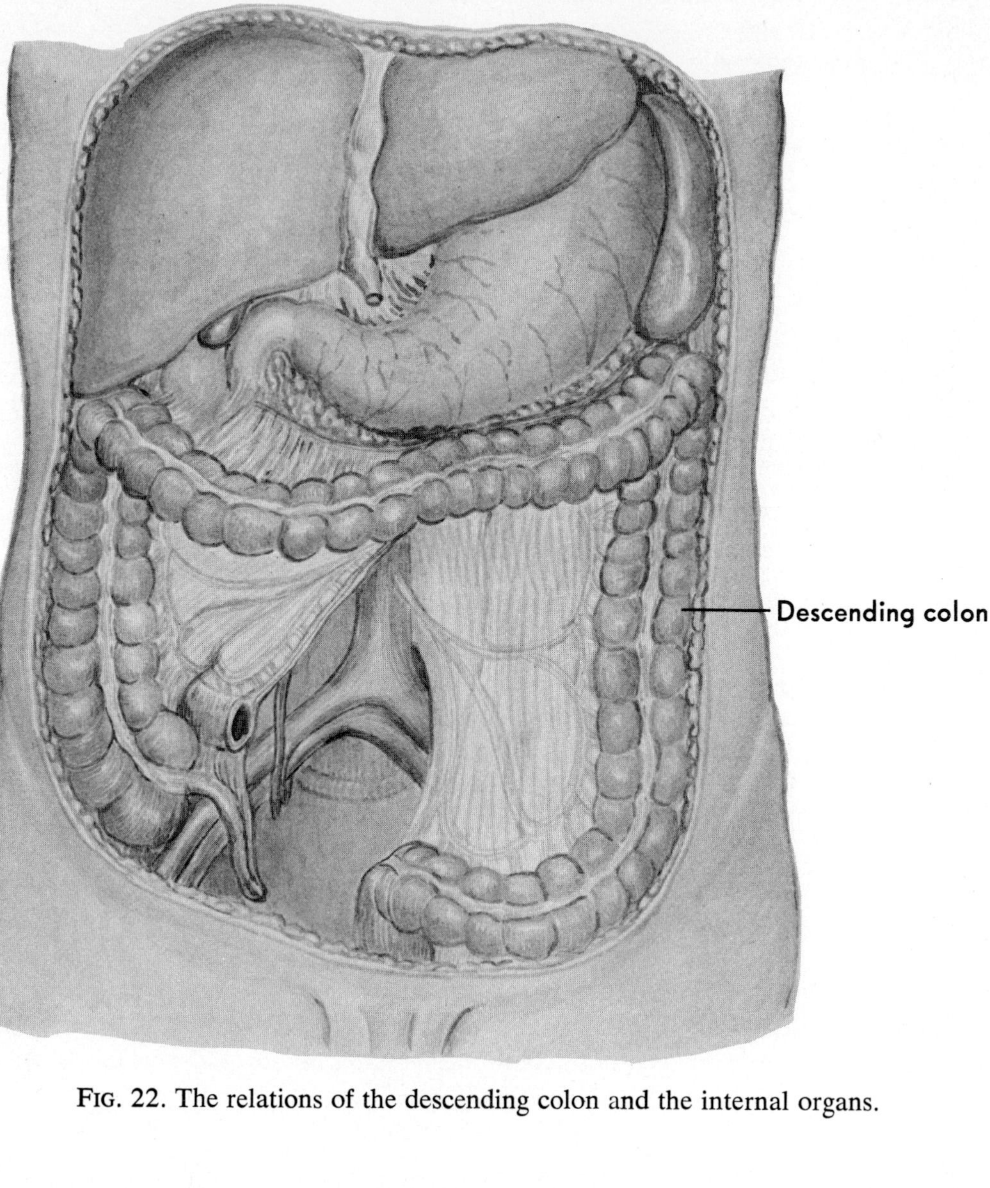

Fig. 22. The relations of the descending colon and the internal organs.

riorly and laterally, while posteriorly it is related to the fascia of the quadratus lumborum in its lumbar segment and the fascia of the iliacus and the psoas muscles in its iliac segment. A definite descending mesocolon has been noted by Treves in 36 out of 100 bodies examined, although Lesskoff noted it only in 16 per cent.

Peritoneal Fold

Only one peritoneal fold is of interest—the persistent descending mesocolon. Despite the presence of a descending mesocolon, the descending colon is less mobile than the ascending colon when a persistent ascending mesocolon is present.

Fixation and Support

The descending colon is supported and fixed in place by: (1) continuity with the splenic flexure above and the pelvic colon below; (2) fixation to the posterior body wall by fusion of its posterior surface; (3) anterolateral investment of peritoneum; (4) its vascular pedicle; and (5) normal intra-abdominal pressure.

PELVIC COLON

Older anatomic usage defines the sig-

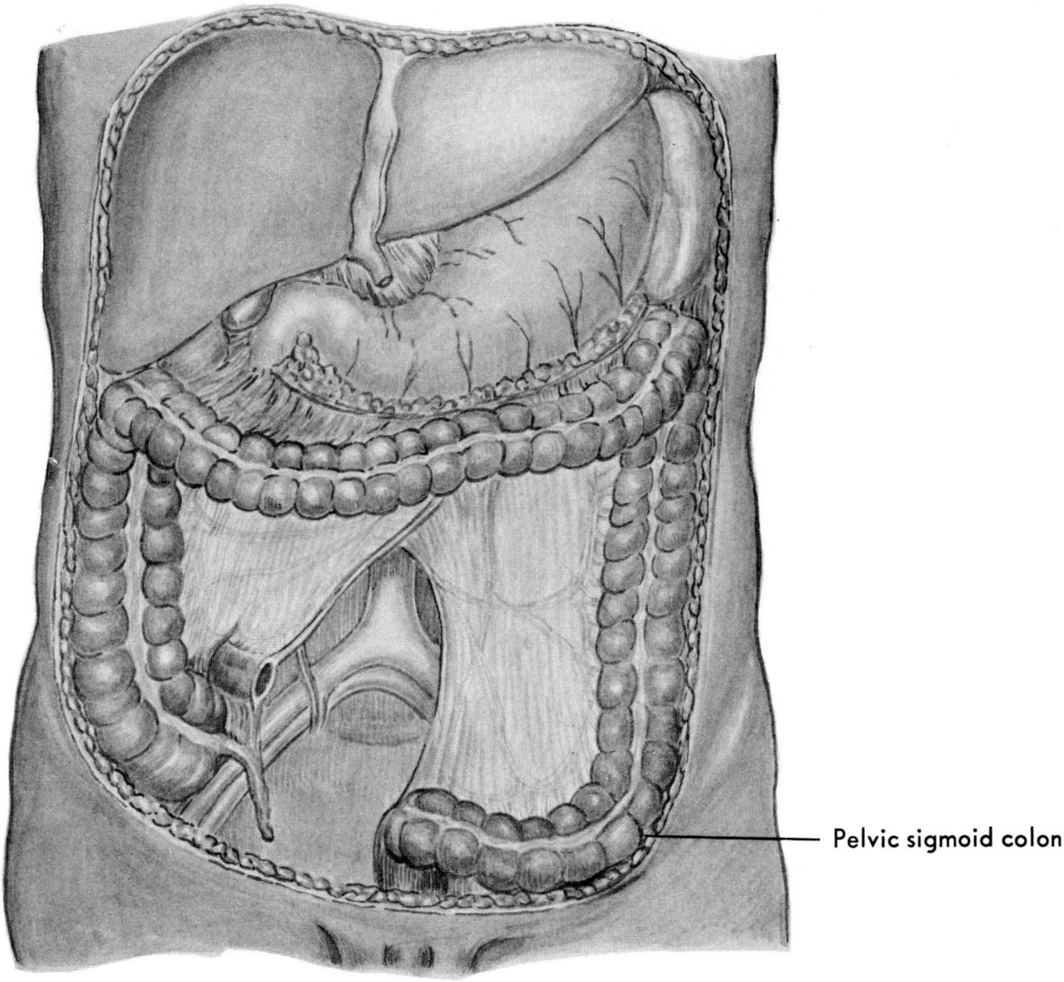

FIG. 23. The relations of the pelvic (sigmoid) colon and the internal organs.

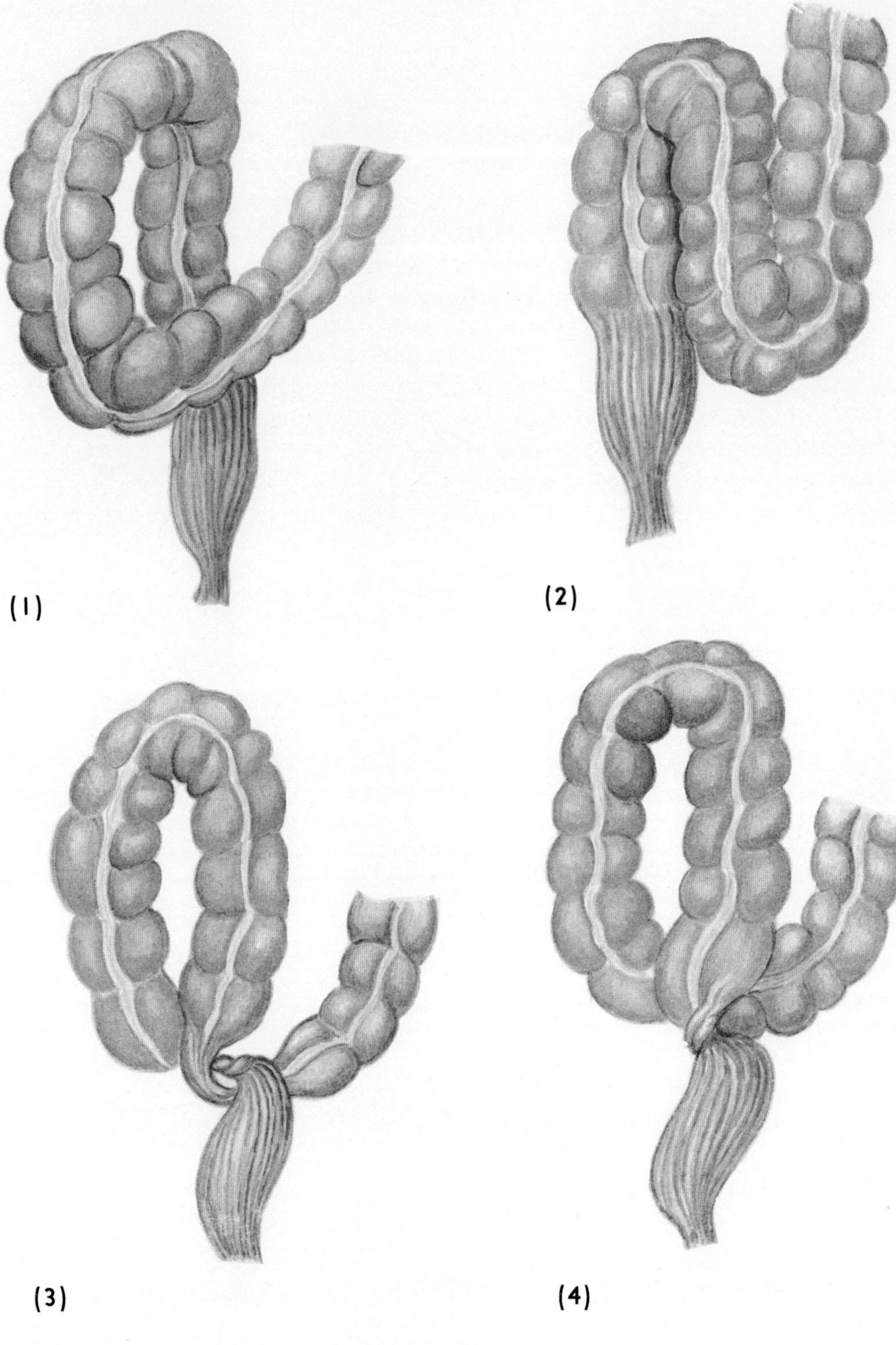

FIG. 24. Various degrees of torsion (redrawn from Brundsgaard). (1) Physiologic volvulus. (2) Long sigmoid. (3) 360° volvulus with torsion and strangulation. (4) Axial torsion in 180° volvulus.

moid colon as extending from the level of the iliac crest down to the region of the rectosigmoid, in the mid-line at the level of the 3rd sacral vertebra. By former usage, it was divided into a fixed iliac segment bound to the iliacus fascia, and a mobile hanging segment by its mesocolon. Clinically, it is better to consider the fixed iliac portion together with the fixed lumbar portion as forming parts of a fixed descending colon, and to consider the pelvic colon as a different segment. The pelvic segment is actually omegoid rather than sigmoid, that is, shaped like omega rather than like sigma. In 7 out of 10 bodies it was found to be omegoid; in only 1 of the remaining 3 (from the original 10 bodies) could it be considered actually sigmoid. Then one body showed it as a straight tube with a short mesocolon, and in the last as 2 parallel loops.

The pelvic colon is almost as long as the transverse colon and has the same mobility. Usually it is 25 to 40 cm. (10 to 16 in.) long, although it may vary from 10 to 90 cm. (4 to 36 in.) in length. If unusually long and mobile, it may be located in the right iliac region and may even touch the diaphragm, which is not unusual in Hirschsprung's disease. If long, it could easily be exteriorized and also may be the frequent site of volvulus. The length and the mobility of the pelvic colon are determined by the length of the mesocolon and the amount of fat in the latter. Over the pelvic mesocolon the appendices epiploicae are most prominent and most numerous; therefore, diverticulosis here is of most frequent occurrence. The taenia coli also tend to spread out gradually toward the more distal portion of the pelvic colon, until at the rectosigmoid, where they fuse again.

Relations

The organ is related to and may be separated by coils of jejuno-ileum from the urinary bladder and the greater omentum anteriorly and the sacrum posteriorly. Behind it passes the left ureter, which may be found at the apex of the intersigmoid fossa. The vessels that supply and drain the rectum run between the leaves of the mesocolon.

Peritoneal Investment

The pelvic colon is invested with peritoneum in its entire extent except for the posterior attachment of the pelvic mesocolon.

Peritoneal Folds and Membranes

The pelvic colon hangs freely by the pelvic mesocolon which is constantly present, although its length varies. As the dorsal mesocolon fuses with the parietal peritoneum, it forms an inverted V-shaped junction with the parietal peritoneum. As a rule, the place of attachment itself runs in an oblique direction. There are 2 limbs to the line of attachment, an ascending (lateral) limb which extends from the middle of the left external iliac artery passing toward the right to the middle of the left common iliac artery, and a descending (medial) limb which extends from here, curving upon itself, toward the left to reach the mid-line at the level of the 3rd sacral segment. It decreases in length from the center toward the ends of the pelvic loop and is fixed at the ends while free in the center, not unlike the disposition of the transverse mesocolon. Out of 20 bodies examined, the pelvic colon had an oblique attachment in 13; it was vertically disposed in 1; present as a single line in 2; and a double line of attachment in the remaining 4 bodies. The intersigmoid fossa is at the apex of the V, where the limbs of the pelvic mesocolon meet.

Only one avascular peritoneal thickening is related to the pelvic colon, the so-called mesosigmoid membrane of Lane. This is found in the iliac fossa, binding the junction of the iliac and the pelvic segments of the colon to the pelvic brim. Lane called this the first and last kink, the first to appear and involving the last part of the bowel. This membrane is homologous to Jackson's membrane on the right side and requires section to mobilize and liberate the pelvic colon.

Fixation and Supports

The pelvic colon is supported and fixed in place by: (1) attachment of the pelvic mesocolon with its contained vessels; (2) continuity to the fixed rectum and the iliac portion of the descending colon; (3) peritoneal investment binding it to the pelvic wall; and (4) normal intra-abdominal pressure.

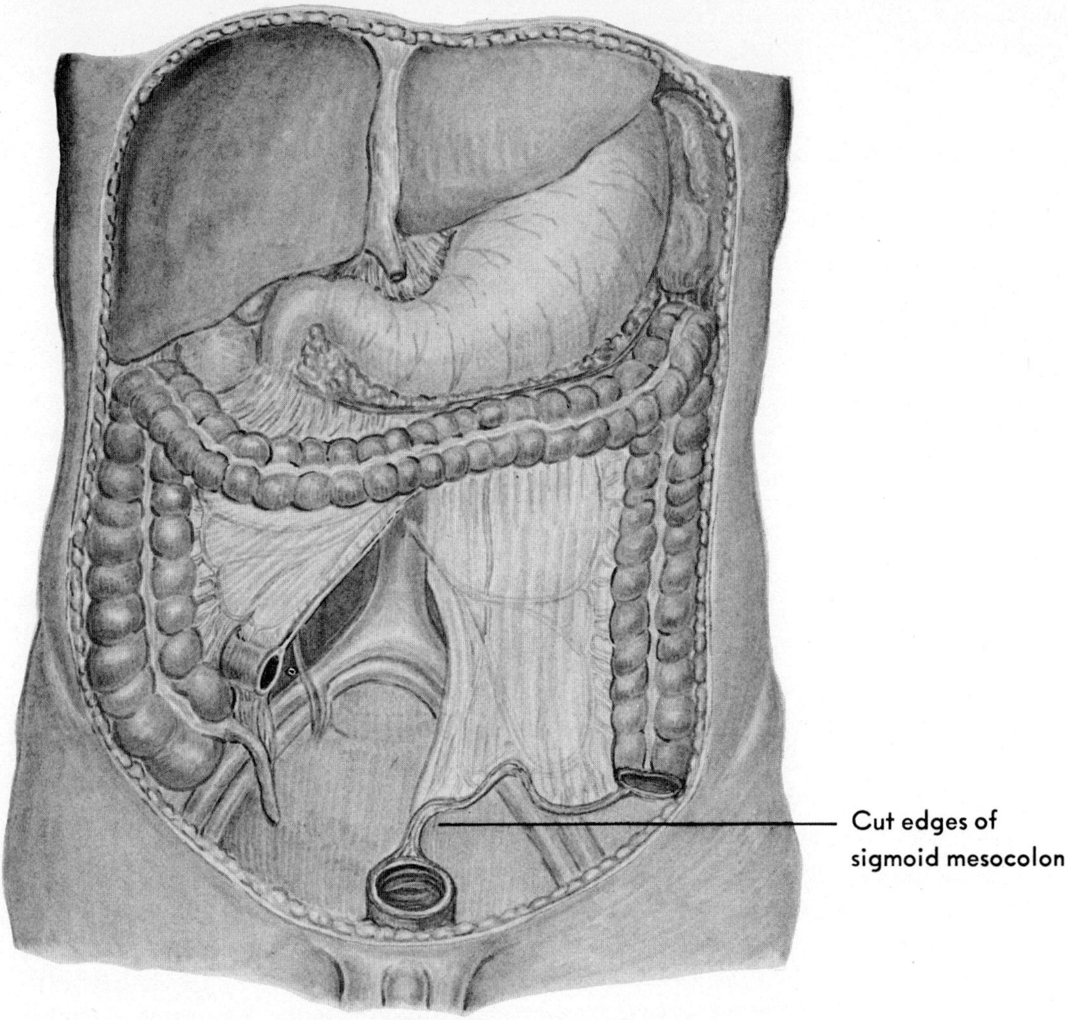

Fig. 25. The mesenteries and their attachments (sigmoid colon).

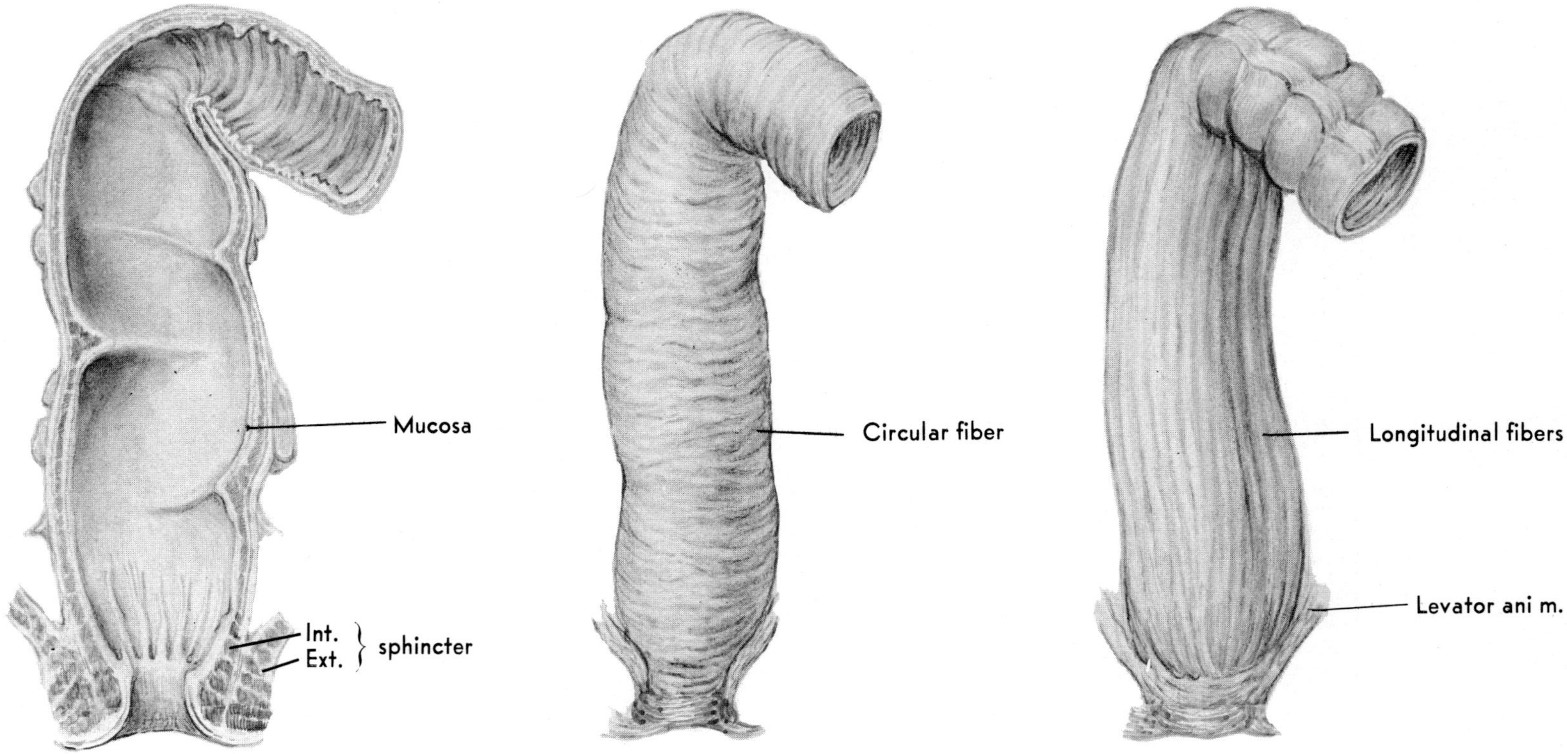

FIG. 26. Longitudinal view of anal canal, rectum and lower sigmoid colon.

RECTOSIGMOID

The precise anatomic location of this indistinctly defined junction between the rectum and the pelvic colon is subject to much discussion. It is called the *recto-sigmoid junction* clinically or the *pelvi-rectal junction* surgically. The lower 2 to 3 cm. of the distal pelvic colon are so intimately related to the upper rectum as regards accessibility, blood supply and lymphatic drainage that clinically this area has been designated rectosigmoid.

Where the colon merges into the rectum certain anatomic features are noted.

1. The peritoneum ceases to invest almost completely the colon; the pelvic mesocolon (mesosigmoid) disappears, and the rectum becomes fused with the sacral wall, and in this part is covered by peritoneum only at the anterior wall and both sides.

2. The bowel becomes fixed at this point, not being provided with a distinct mesocolon, like the mobile pelvic colon.

3. The 3 distinct bands of longitudinal muscle fuse again, so that a more-or-less complete coat encircles the bowel, although the layer seems to be thicker and more prominent anteriorly than posteriorly.

4. The appendices epiploicae become less prominent and may even be entirely absent.

5. The saccular haustrations are lost, because the longitudinal muscle again forms a complete coat of the bowel.

6. The superior hemorrhoidal vessels leave the pelvic colon to lie behind the rectum and divide into 2 terminal branches that course alongside the rectum.

7. The inconstant diminution of caliber (to one third of the cecum) and a variable degree of angulation and fixation may be present.

8. Internally, the rugose mucosa of the pelvic colon, which is converted into longitudinal folds in its distal extremity, is replaced by the smooth mucous membrane of the rectum. There is also an increased vascularity, looseness and distensibility of the rectum.

These anatomic features are generally noted in the mid-line, opposite the 3rd segment of the sacrum.

RECTUM

Literally, the rectum is a straight tube. The earliest anatomic dissections were made on animals, usually pigs, in which that segment of the bowel was straight, and originally rectum. Since it led to the anus, it was named after the latter—proctos. Later, the term persisted because the organ is fixed in the mid-line; thus, when seen anteroposteriorly, it presented a straight vertical line on the sacrum down to the coccyx.

Extent

Strictly speaking, the rectum extends from the rectosigmoid junction to the termination of its circular muscle as the internal sphincter of the anal canal. Then the latter would necessarily be included in the anatomic scope of the rectum. Clinically, however, the distal boundary is taken at the anorectal line or junction, or where it pierces the pelvic diaphragm, a point about 2 cm. in front of the coccyx. Others consider the apex of the prostate gland or the lower fourth of the posterior vaginal wall as the boundary. The rectum varies in length as well as in diameter. Usually, it is 12 to 15 cm. long, although it seems to be longer if the rectovesical or the rectouterine space is deeper as in children or in those with persistent cul-de-sac. There is variation as well in diameter and distensibility. Large foreign bodies, as beer bottles, could easily be accommodated by the capacious rectal ampulla. The peritoneum is intimately attached at the rectosigmoid junction, but as the rectum descends it becomes more loosely attached, thereby allowing expansion of the rectum when needed.

Division

Time and again, the rectum has been variously divided into clinical and anatomic areas. Sappey considered the rectum to start from the left iliac synchrondrosis, which is now considered as part of the pelvic colon. He divided the rectum into a superior, a middle and an inferior part, the superior corresponding to the terminal part of the pelvic colon, the middle to the rectal ampulla, and the inferior to the anal canal. The ampulla is the dilated portion of the rectum lying in the pelvis and covered by peritoneum in its lateral and anterior surfaces. Tuttle described a sacrococcygeal and a prostatic rectum, while Waldeyer referred to a pelvic portion and a perineal or sphincteric portion. Others consider the rectum in relation to its peritoneal investment, that is, an upper intraperitoneal rectum and a lower intraperitoneal rectum. The wide upper ampullary portion is the widest part of the bowel and is more marked in children, multipara and those with pelvic relaxation. It is bounded by the rectosigmoid above and the anal canal below, although others would place the lower limit at the level of the second rectal valve.

Curves

The rectum curves in both anteroposterior and lateral directions. The anteroposterior curves are: (1) convex backwards as the rectum fits into the sacral hollow, and (2) convex forward where it joins the anal canal, with the anococcygeal body at its junction. In the lateral view, it has 3 curves or flexures. The upper and the lower curves are concave toward the left, while the middle is concave toward the right. These flexures become exaggerated when the rectum is distended, and they correspond to the attachment of the rectal valves. Considering the location of these flexures and curves, one may imagine the rectum to be more or less a spiral tube which turns first to the right, then across the mid-line, to the left and finally proceeds to the mid-line again, where it becomes the anal canal.

Relations

Anteriorly, the pelvic rectum is related to a varying length of the terminal part of the pelvic colon, depending upon the mobility and the length of the pelvic mesocolon. Loops of the jejuno-ileum and even the vermiform appendix may fill the pelvis and thus be related to the rectum anteriorly. In front are the uterus in the female and the urinary bladder in the male.

Below the peritoneal reflection it is related anteriorly to, and separated by, Denonvilliers' rectovesical fascia from the interdeferent triangle or interampullary triangle on the posterior surface of the urinary bladder; the prostate gland at whose apex is attached the rectourethral muscle of Roux; seminal vesicles, the vas deferens, and the juxtavesical portion of both ureters. In the female, the relations are the uterus directly in front and the adnexae a little to each side. Because of the free and mobile distal pelvic colon, tumors and intussusception of the latter may be felt by ballottement through the rectal wall. Hence, what at times may be felt as a growth in the upper rectum may

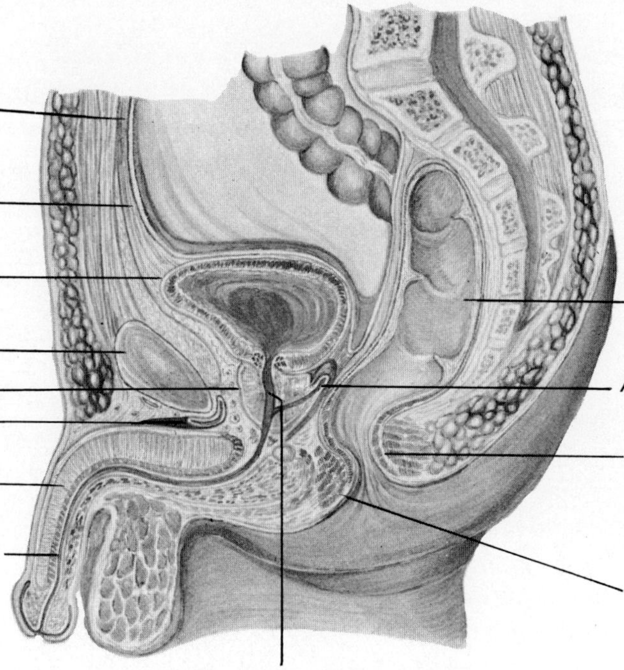

FIG. 27. Midsagittal section of the pelvic viscera (male).

actually be a tumor arising from the distal pelvic colon.

In pelvic appendicitis, tenderness could be elicited by rectal examination. Similarly, masses of ileocecal intussusception may be palpated through the rectum, especially in children. The urinary bladder may be tapped, and stones in it palpated through the base of the interdeferent triangle.

The normal prostate gland may also be easily felt, and change in its size, consistency, and surface may be easily detected. The seminal vesicles may be felt, when distended like short, small Vienna sausages which extend like rabbit ears. Section of Denonvilliers' prostatoperineal or rectovesical fascia just above the rectovesical fold will open the prostatoperineal space of Denonvilliers bordered by the rectourethralis muscle, attaining importance in perineal prostatectomy. This is also called the *retroprostatic cleavage space of Proust,* and is an avascular cleavage plane between the rectum and the prostate gland.

In infections involving Cowper's bulbourethral glands, tenderness may be elicited in front of the level of the pelvic diaphragm. The rectovesical fascia prevents reciprocal spread of cancer of the prostate and the rectum. Impacted stones in the juxtavesical ureters may be palpated rectally. Urethral sounds may be aided in passing through the pelvic diaphragm with a finger in the rectum. In the female, displacements of the uterus and the direction of the cervix may be detected.

To the uninitiated, the cervix, when felt rectally, may be mistaken for a small polypoid tumor. Owing to the proximity between the vagina and the rectum, fecal impactions may be partially expelled with the aid of a stripping finger in the vagina.

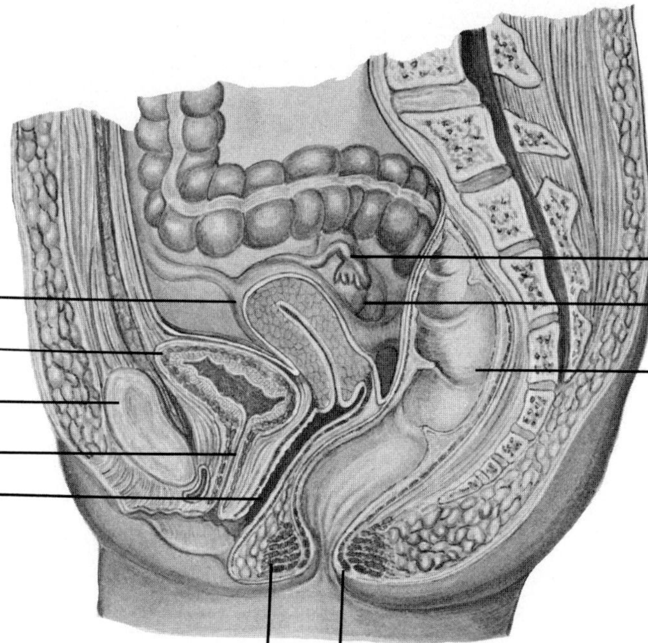

FIG. 28. Midsagittal section of the pelvic viscera (female).

Furthermore, in cases of anorectal stenosis, digital examination of the rectal wall may be done through the vagina. The progress of labor may be traced by periodic rectal examinations. Owing to the relation to the bottom of the cul-de-sac of Douglas, exploratory puncture of the latter may be done through a proctotomy in males and a colpotomy in females. Metastases dropping into the cul-de-sac or rectal peritoneal shelf from growths in the pancreas, the gallbladder, the ascending colon, the breast and the stomach may also be detected rectally.

Laterally may be found the ischial spine, which serves as a landmark for the progress of labor. Through the rectal wall and the pelvic diaphragm may be felt the greater sciatic foramen, the piriformis muscle, the gluteal vessels and nerves, the internal pudendal vessels and nerves, the sciatic nerve, the posterior femoral cutaneous nerve, the nerve to the quadratus femoris and the obturator internus. The internal iliac artery and its branches are also related to the rectum laterally. The ovaries and the ends of the fallopian tubes are also located laterally. Rectal tenderness may be elicited in salpingitis and ectopic pregnancy. When the rectum is distended, it is related directly to the piriformis muscle and the left sacral plexus posterolaterally.

Owing to the number of nerves which lie lateral to the rectum, they could very easily be involved in cancer of the rectum. For this reason, severe pain in the sacral area is not unusual in these instances. The nerve sheaths themselves have been proved to be a route for metastatic spread of rectal cancer. Because of the reflection of the peritoneum, it lies in contact with the pyramidalis muscle, the gluteal, the internal pudendal and the sciatic vessels as well as the sciatic, the lumbodorsal and the sacral nerves. Laterally and directed posteriorly are also found Jonnesco's lateral ligaments of the pelvic rectum (the lateral rectal stalks), suspensory ligaments of the rectum, which represent prolongation of the endopelvic fascia with condensation of areolar tissue about the middle hemorrhoidal vessels and the nervi erigentes, also referred to as the middle hemorrhoidal neurovascular stalk. In the female, this may be subdivided into a large posterolateral retrorectal and a small anterolateral rectovaginal component. They are attached to the lower two thirds of the rectum and are supposed to help support the rectum in place; in the male they also help to support the bladder and the prostate. These lateral ligaments must be sectioned in order to liberate or completely mobilize the rectum. A large middle hemorrhoidal artery or numerous small arteries may be present and may require ligation. Recently, some anatomists have felt that in these instances, the areolar tissue can give little support, and the support has been attributed to the middle hemorrhoidal vessels.

Posteriorly are found the superior hemorrhoidal vessels of which the artery is more intimately in contact with the rectal wall. Further back lies the sacrum and the coccyx, with the median sacral vessels, the sacral vessels and nerves, the hypogastric plexus in the retrorectal or presacral space in between. Tumors, especially cysts, may be located here as remnants of the postanal gut. More lateral than directly posterior are the piriformis, the coccygeus and the levator ani muscles, separated from the rectum by the sympathetic trunk, the lateral sacral vessels and the nerves and the coccygeal nerves. Enlarged hypogastric nodes may be detected posterolaterally.

Peritoneal Investment

The peritoneum does not cover the entire rectum. In the upper part the peritoneum covers the anterior and the lateral parts of the rectum and forms the mesorectum, which is contiguous with the pelvic mesocolon. In the middle part it covers only the anterior surface from which it is reflected in front as the rectovesical fold to the urinary bladder in the male and the rectouterine fold onto the uterus in the female. The third part is wholly infraperitoneal and is not clothed with peritoneum. Instead, the lower part is covered by (1) an inner cellular sheath adherent to the rectum, which forms part of the lateral ligaments, together with (2) an outer fibrous sheath, the fascia propria arising from the sacrum and connected with the fascia of either prostate or vagina. The peritoneum is reflected from each side of the anterior part of the rectum to the posterolateral wall of the pelvis, forming the pararectal fossae. This line of peritoneal reflection corresponds to the middle rectal valve of Houston inside the rectal lumen. In the newborn, the peritoneum lies low, covering the posterior surface of the urinary bladder, the seminal vesicles and the prostate gland. It may even reach the pelvic floor, which is the level at the 4th to the 5th month of intrauterine life. Soon after birth, these layers fuse to form the rectovesical or prostatoperineal fascia of Denonvillier or Tyrell's fascia. If nonfusion persists, a perineal hernia or vaginal enterocoele may develop.

Fixation and Supports

The rectum has no mesentery of its

own. What is sometimes termed the mesorectum is the condensation of the areolar tissue about the superior hemorrhoidal vessels that lie directly posterior and also postlateral to the rectum, containing it further back to the pelvic wall.

The rectum is held in place by: (1) continuity with the colon above and the anal canal below; (2) peritoneal investment fixing it against the posterior pelvic wall; (3) mesorectum (which refers to the areolar tissue on the posterior aspect of the upper part of the rectum which contains the superior hemorrhoidal vessels) and probably some support from the pelvic mesocolon; (4) the levator diaphragm upon which the rectum partially rests and with whose fibers the longitudinal muscle interdigitates; (5) Waldeyer's fascia, which is a reflection of the sacral fascia at the level of the sacrococcygeal articulation and encloses the superior hemorrhoidal vessels and suspends the ampulla; (6) the lateral ligaments, although the degree and the amount of support that these structures could offer has been questioned; (7) Denonvilliers' fascia and its homolog in the female; and (8) the pelvic diaphragm.

Variations

In children the rectum is straight, more vertical, and more tubular than in the adult, because the flexures and Houston's rectal valves are not developed until after infancy. Furthermore, owing to the incomplete development of the pelvis in children, the rectum is more an abdominal organ than in adults. The presence of lax connective tissue between the mucosa and the muscular coats is responsible for the unusual mobility of the former upon the latter and the propensity to prolapse in children if they develop diarrhea.

Internal Structure of the Rectum

The rectal mucosa appears pink to dark red, owing to the vascular capillary network that shows through. It is smooth and may even have a velvety appearance, owing to the numerous tiny pits of the crypts of Lieberkühn. These crypts are larger and deeper in the rectum (0.7 mm.) than in the colon (0.45 mm.). In a few instances distinct pitting may be noted. At times the submucosal lymphatic aggregates may be large enough to be prominent on the surface and even be mistaken for adenomas or mammillations. The rectal lumen is often empty and its wall thrown into transverse folds. These folds straighten out when the rectum distends. There is a fair degree of mobility of the rectal mucosa over the submucosa, although the mobility is more marked in infants and children. The inner circular layer in its distal extremity becomes rolled and thickened, serving as the internal sphincter which is found overlapping the upper two thirds of the anal canal. The longitudinal coat has its fibers interdigitating with those of the levator ani, forming the combined longitudinal muscle of the rectum. This combined muscle then splits into numerous fibroelastic extensions between the anorectal sphincters and is finally attached to the superficial fascia of the perianal skin. The tunica serosa of the infraperitoneal portion of the rectum is actually loose areolar tissue. This loose areolar tissue allows the rectal ampulla to distend much beyond any portion of the colon.

Rectal Valves

In the course of proctoscopy one usually sees 3 prominent crescentic, horizontal or obliquely disposed semilunar folds—the rectal valves of Houston. They vary in size, thickness and number. They are usually 3, occasionally 10; at times 4 or even 5 may be present; and in not a few cases none at all may be observed.

They consist of mucosa, submucosa with the greater part formed by the circular muscle of the rectum, thus differing from the valvulae conniventes of the small bowel which are only mucosal folds. Owing to their circular muscle content, their internal position corresponds to the concavity of the lateral flexures of the rectum, upper and lower on the left, and the middle on the right. They serve an unknown function; probably they help support the fecal column and provide a spiral motion to the fecal mass as it is expelled during defecation.

These valves may be altogether absent, especially in those with chronic constipation, in which case the rectal wall appears rugose, with many transverse folds, not unlike the vaginal wall.

They may only be short folds, although they may be so prominent as to extend across half of the circumference of the rectum.

There are usually 3 valves corresponding to the 3 flexures, of which the second is the most prominent. This second valve, which is found at the right side, is often referred to as Kolrausch's transverse fold

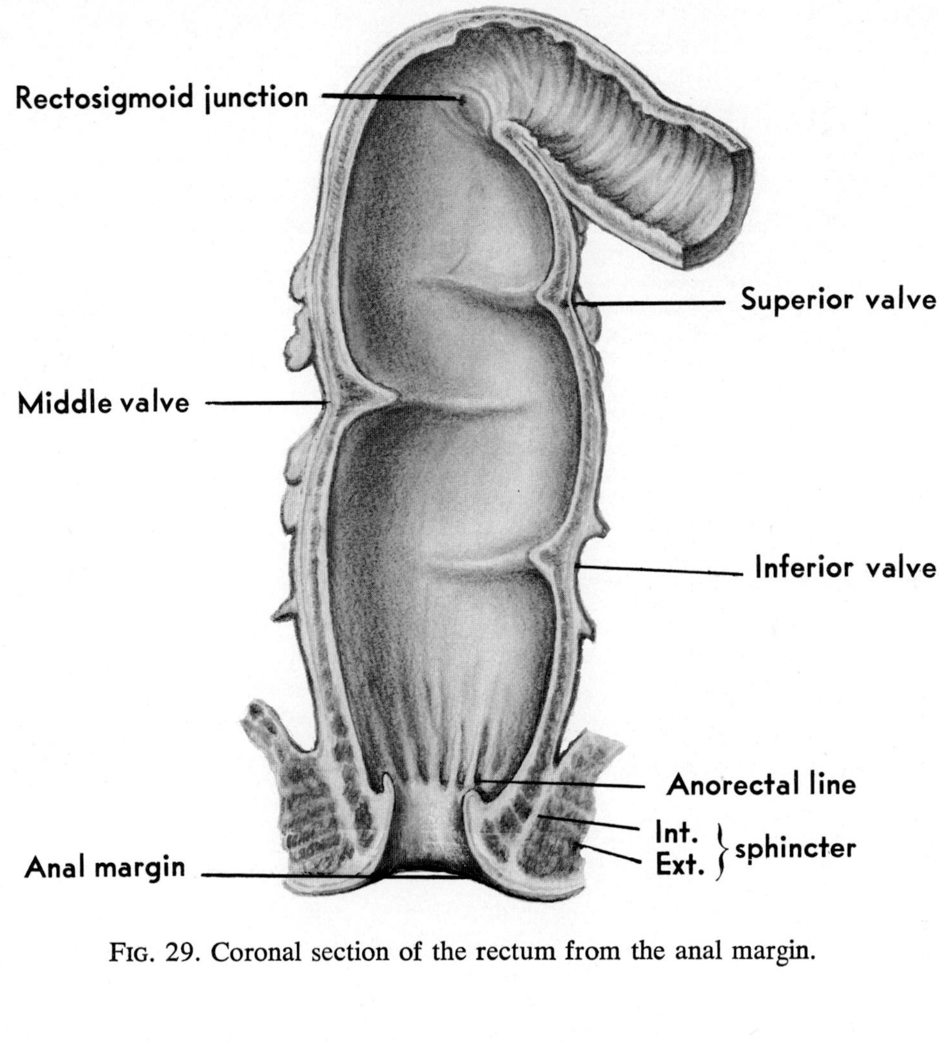

FIG. 29. Coronal section of the rectum from the anal margin.

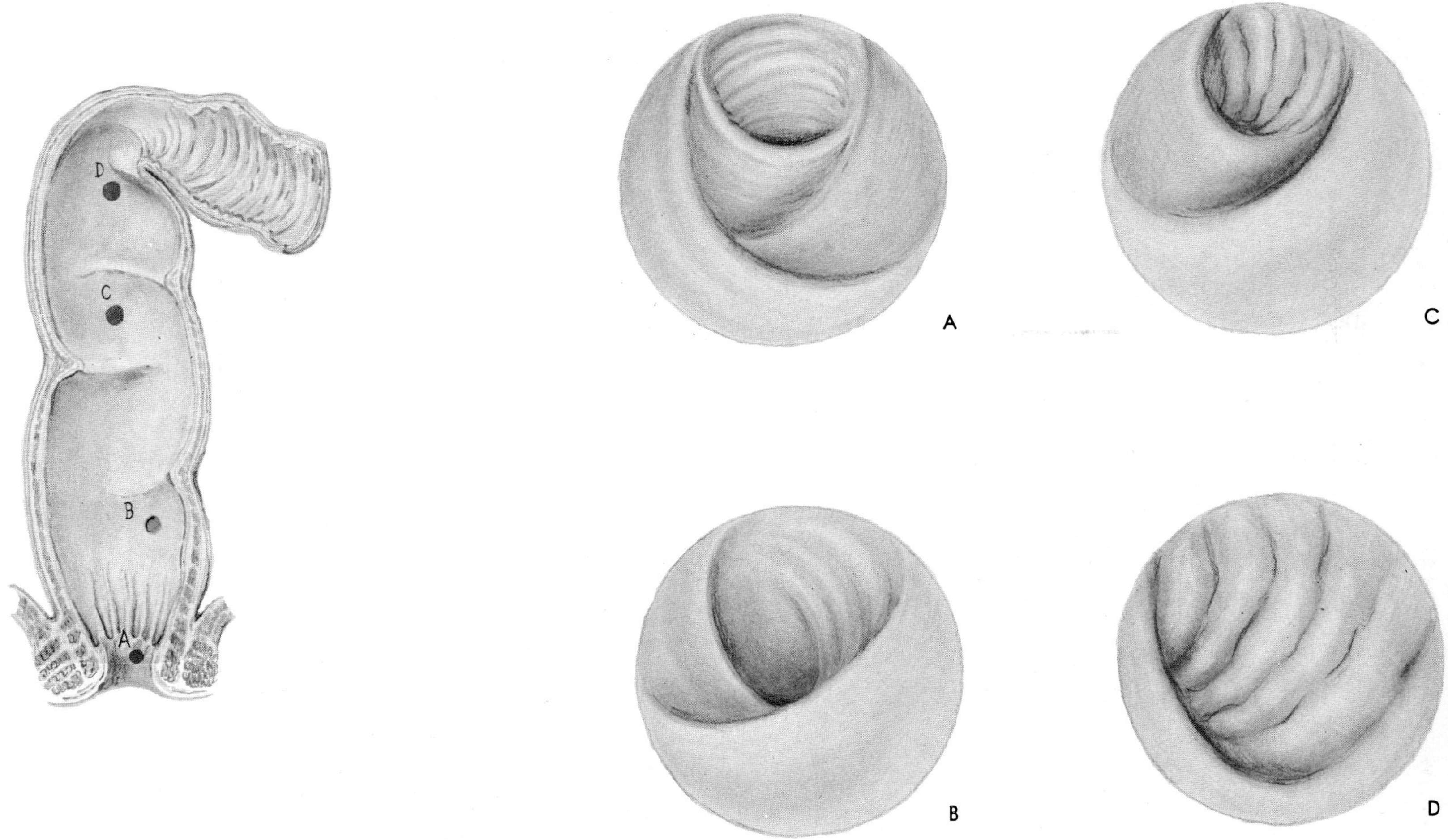

FIG. 30. Proctoscopic views of the anal canal, the rectum and the sigmoid colon.

of the rectum and lies at the level of the peritoneal reflection. Kolrausch's fold is particularly important because at this level there appears to be a definite boundary of the lymphatics of the upper and the lower halves of the rectum and the anal canal. It is also this valve which will frequently prevent the easy passage of the rectal tube. Any valve may hide above it small lesions like ulcers and adenomas; therefore, the valves should be smoothed out during proctoscopy. Normally, these valves have a thin edge; if the edge appears rounded this is taken as evidence of edema. They may also retract, due to previous disease and ulceration, which may be indicated by roughening of the surface. Because of the presence of circular muscle in these valves, especially in the prominent second valve, the latter was once thought to possess sphincteric function and was referred to as the superior sphincter (Nelaton, Velpeau) or third anal sphincter (Hyrtl). This was also called the detrusor faecium (Chadwick) because the muscular elements were believed to expel the feces during defecation. These valves have also been described and studied by Henle, Sappey, Otis, van Buren, Kelsey, Quenu and Hartmann, etc. In case there are more than 3 valves, they are arranged one after the other as they arise from oposite lateral walls.

Surgical Considerations: Proctosigmoidoscopy

Ordinarily, this procedure is carried out in the office and for all intents and purposes should be a part of a general physical examination. The importance of this procedure can never be overemphasized and many times constitutes the most valuable diagnostic procedure. It should always precede a barium enema. The success of the examination is contingent upon a clean, well-prepared bowel and to the effectiveness of the "vocal anesthesia" which the examiner gives to the patient.

The rectum is often examined with the patient in the inverted position, using special examining tables that can be flexed or broken in the middle, corresponding to the level of the hips. In this position, the intestines gravitate toward the diaphragm, emptying the rectovaginal or rectovesical pouch, thereby relieving pressure on the sigmoid. Furthermore, the rectum could dilate with one atmospheric pressure, and this position is easier for the introduction of the examining finger or any special instrument. Usually, patients can be maintained comfortably in this position for long periods.

Digital examination of the anal region should be performed first to determine the general direction and caliber of the anal canal and the lower rectum, whether it would be feasible to use the standard ⅝-inch sigmoidoscope, and to detect any existing pathology in the general area. Should a painful lesion be present, a smaller caliber instrument and the use of a topical anesthetic might be indicated, which will add to the comfort of the patient and in turn provide maximal cooperation and unhurried thorough examination.

The sigmoidoscope is introduced with the right hand, keeping in mind the angle between the direction of the anal canal and the direction of the rectum. The instrument is aimed in the direction of the umbilicus, and as soon as the resistance presented by the anus is overcome, the instrument is held firmly by the left hand with the left elbow firmly rested on the left buttock, and the obturator is removed. This is a very important point to remember because perforation or laceration of the rectum may occur if the flange is thrust forward in overcoming the natural resistance encountered in removing the obturator. From then on the instrument is advanced by direct visualization of the lumen for clues to the lumen ahead. This part of the procedure may be facilitated by the introduction of air into the rectum, but this should be allowed to escape since it is liable to cause discomfort to the patient.

The valves of Houston are seen as folds projecting into the lumen. The most constant fold is the middle valve located in the right anterior wall, 11 cm. (4½ in.) from the anal margin. This marks the level of the peritoneal reflection and also marks the boundary between the lymphatics of the upper and the lower rectum and the anal canal. The rectosigmoid junction is marked by narrowing of the lumen, 3.5 cm. (1¼ in.) above the superior rectal valve.

While the sigmoid generally passes to the left, the examiner should be alert for an occasional sigmoid that passes to the right. This area is sometimes referred to as a blind alley; and in order to advance the scope it may be necessary to withdraw and advance it again. Pain and variable degrees of discomfort are experienced by the patient and may be referred to the stomach.

Having successfully passed the sigmoidoscope the usual distance of 25 cm. (10 in.), examination, diagnosis and possibly biopsy of a lesion is made as the instrument is withdrawn. Since the field of vision through the scope is limited, manipulation through the entire circumference is made in order to visualize all its aspects, paying particular attention to the numerous folds of the sigmoid and the mucosa behind the rectal valves.

Proctosigmoidoscopic examination in infants and children is carried out in the same manner, using the same length instrument except when pathologic processes and anomalies are present. From the technical standpoint, insertion and passage of the instrument may be easier in children than in adults because the rectum and the sigmoid colon are straight, more nearly vertical, and more tubular, and the rectal valves and flexures are not well developed until after infancy.

Rectal biopsy is accomplished with the use of a biopsy forceps. The site of biopsy may be fulgurated for control of bleeding.

Rectal biopsy performed for diagnosis of Hirschsprung's disease deserves special consideration. It should be made 2 to 3 cm. from the anorectal line and must include both longitudinal and circular muscle layers so that the presence or the absence of ganglion cells in the myenteric plexus can be examined. A portion of the rectal mucosa and submucosa may be included to determine the presence or the absence of ganglion cells in Meissner's submucosal plexus. Normally, the ganglion cells in the latter plexus are difficult to demonstrate; therefore, absence is not diagnostic of the entity. The purpose of obtaining the biopsy at the level of 2 to 3 cm. above the anorectal line is to include the biopsy incision in the bowel to be resected.

ANORECTAL JUNCTION

The terminal portion of the rectum becomes angulated backward due to the pull of the puborectalis muscle as the latter encloses the anal canal. The anal canal begins at the apex of the prostate gland at the level of the levator ani muscle and is directed backward and downward, ending in the anal opening below.

Significance

The anorectal junction marks where the

entodermal rectum telescopes into the ectodermal anal canal, forming a serrated border, called also the dentate line (the anal papillae appear like small teats), pectinate line (the anal papillae and the rectal columns have a comblike arrangement), the anorectal line, or mucocutaneous junction. This region represents the dividing line between the visceral and the somatic nervous systems, the portal and the caval circulations, and the visceral and the somatic lymphatics.

Internal Structure

Internally, the anorectal junction presents numerous anatomic features. At the lower part of the rectum are found 5 to 10 slender pyramidal foldings (about 2 cm. long, more or less) of the mucosa covering localized condensations of the longitudinal terminal branch of the superior hemorrhoidal artery, and tributary vein for the superior hemorrhoidal plexus. These are called the columns of Morgagni and have been described earlier as the pillars of Glisson. These columns are effaced during distention of the rectum. The furrows between the longitudinal ridges are called the anorectal sinuses, rectal sinuses above the anorectal line and anal sinuses below the anorectal line. The bases of two adjacent columns are joined by a semilunar membranous fold called the anal valve (of Cloquet, Portal, Morgagni), the free edge of which projects inward and upward. The rectal sinuses between the rectal valves end in shallow blind cup-shaped anal sinuses or funnel-shaped anal crypts, 3 to 5 mm. deep, behind the anal valves. These blind pouches are called the crypts of Morgagni or the saccules of Horner and are also referred to as anal pockets. Projecting upward from the free edge of the anal valve

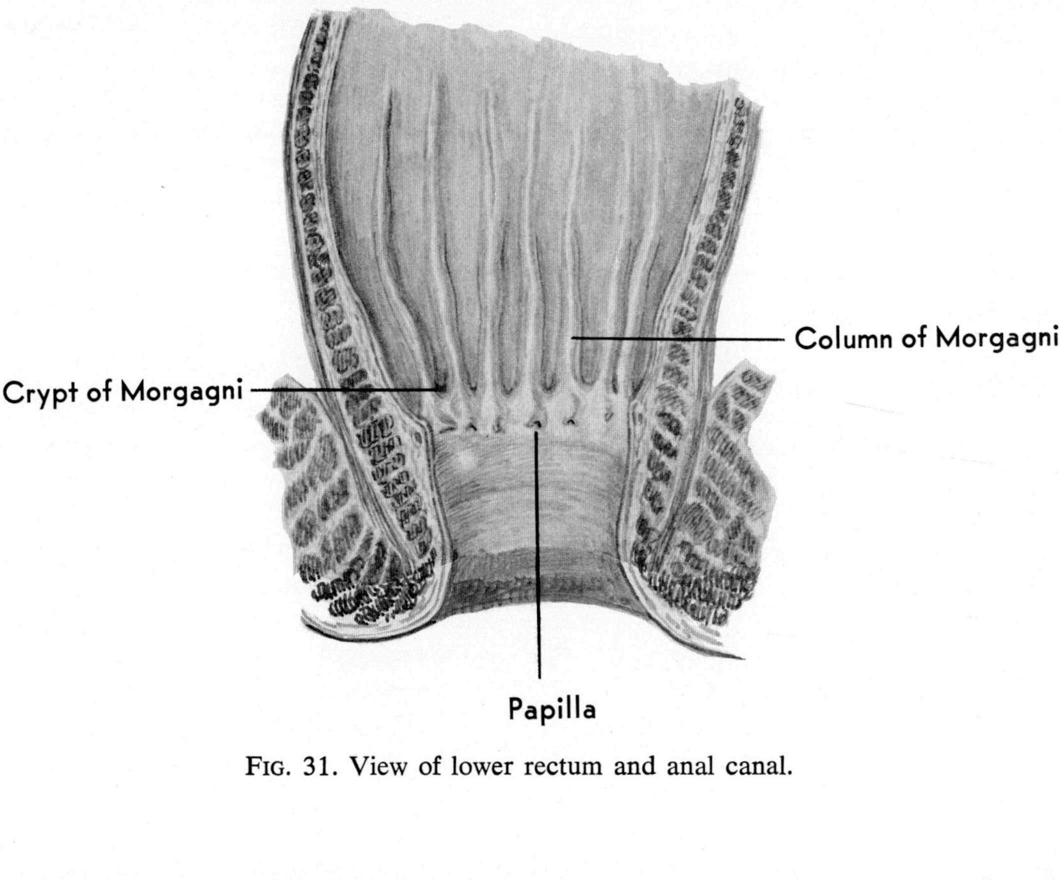

FIG. 31. View of lower rectum and anal canal.

or direct from the base of the rectal column may be found a rudimentary conical, nipplelike process called the anal papilla of Morgagni.

Clinical Importance

The anal crypts are important clinically because into them empty the deep intramuscular or anorectal glands which have been shown to play a role in the etiopathogenesis of nonspecific infections of the rectum and the canal. In addition, they store mucus which is poured out during defecation and helps lubricate the descending fecal mass. Tearing of the anal valves could serve as a focus for invasion by pathogens. The anal papillae may become enlarged, due to lymphatic obstruction from inflammatory processes in the surrounding tissue.

ANAL CANAL

The terminal portion of the digestive tract is a short ectodermal derivative called the anal canal. It varies in length from 1.5 to 4 cm. and can dilate to 3 cm. or more during defecation. Due to angulation of the anal canal, its anterior wall is 1 cm. longer than the posterior wall. It extends from the fixed anorectal line above to the inconstant anocutaneous line below. The canal may be lengthened by hypertrophy of the internal sphincter and by contraction of the subcutaneous portion of the external sphincter. When the anal canal is closed, the external sphincter envelops the internal sphincter, but when the canal is open the lower margin of the internal sphincter becomes proximal to the lower margin of the external sphincter. Normally, the anal canal is closed with its lateral walls in apposition, and dilates only during the passage of gas or the evacuation of stool.

Internal Structure

Being an ectodermal derivative, the anal canal is lined by skin. The upper third is lined by modified epithelium. It is adherent to the underlying tissue and is tedious to dissect out in operations on the rectum with preservation of the anorectal sphincters. The lower two thirds of the anal canal is lined by skin and has the usual cutaneous appendages like sweat glands, sebaceous glands and hair follicles. Beyond the anal verge, true skin is found also. Upon anoscopy, the anoderm is seen as a thin, slightly bluish membrane, stretched as it is over the external hemorrhoidal plexus, which imparts to the former a darker and redder congested appearance compared with the lighter pink of the rectal mucosa.

At the junction of the upper and the middle thirds of the anal canal may be noted a bluish line, better designated as a slight depression, where the external sphincter envelops the internal sphincter. This corresponds to the so-called white line of Hilton or the intersphincteric line of Hibshman. The upper third of the anal canal between the anorectal line and Hilton's line is referred to as the pecten by Stroud. Usually it marks the extent of the anorectal glands and ducts in the subepithelial areolar tissue of the anal canal and contains smooth muscle fibers, possibly extensions of the muscularis mucosae which have been described as surrounding the anal canal. This muscular ring is referred to as the orbicularis ani by Smith. Fine and Lawes have described a musculus submucosa ani, which is a conglomeration of smooth muscle fibers from Kolrausch's sustentator tunicae mucosae (well-developed muscularis mucosae of the terminal rectum) and cranial extensions of the conjoined longitudinal muscle bundle.

Spasm of this muscle band has been thought to simulate pectinosis. Recurrent inflammation involving the anorectal gland and duct system results in fibrous replacement in this area. This state is called pectenosis, and the definite band formed is called pecten band. Section of this band has been termed pectenotomy by some surgeons.

While the anoderm covers the lower two thirds of the anal canal, it is not as loose as the rectal mucosa. Ending in the anoderm and the terminal rectum are the receptors of the defecation reflex, and thus the anal canal and the terminal rectum should be spared and left intact if the defecation reflex is to be preserved. It has no peritoneum, and its adventitial coat is closely related all around to a muscular cylinder formed by the anal sphincter and the levator ani muscle. On each side are found the two para-anal spaces, the ischioanal spaces, more improperly termed ischiorectal spaces. Behind it is the fibromuscular anococcygeal body which separates it from the coccyx. Anteriorly, it is separated by areolar tissue from the membranous portion or the bulb of the urethra in males, while the fibromuscular perineal body separates it from the vagina in females.

Fixation and Support

The anal canal is supported and fixed in place by: (1) the anorectal sphincters around it; (2) anococcygeal body behind it; (3) perineal body in front; (4) pelvic diaphragm at which level it takes origin; and (5) continuity with the rectum above.

Anorectal Sphincters

The direct sphincteric action at the anal canal is effected by a muscular cylinder which includes the internal anal sphincter, the longitudinal muscle band of the rectum, the external anal sphincter, and the levator ani muscle. The internal anal sphincter consists of smooth muscle and represents an aggregate of the lowermost fibers of the circular muscle of the rectal wall. It is an inch long and encloses the upper two thirds of the anal canal, where its lower end may be felt just below the subcutaneous portion of the external sphincter. It serves to empty the anal canal completely after the passage of the fecal mass, although some believe that the muscle has no share in the preservation of continence.

The longitudinal muscle coat of the rectum is prolonged and extended beyond the anal canal and forms part of the muscular cylinder around it. It is thinner laterally but is broader anteriorly and posteriorly. Above the anorectal angle, the longitudinal muscle sends two slips attached to the upper part of the perineal body, the superior and the inferior bundles of the rectourethralis muscle of Roux. These must be cut before the plane between the prostate gland and the rectum can be reached. Posteriorly, a flat longitudinal muscle band extends from the coccyx to the pelvic brim, the bilateral rectococcygeus muscle of Treitz and Kolrausch. It is prolonged between the internal anal sphincters and interdigitates with muscular fascicles from the puborectalis portion of the levator ani muscle, at the same time receiving fibrotendinous extensions from the superior layers of the pelvic diaphragm. All these elements finally form the fibromuscular sheath of the rectum variously called the longitudinal muscle or tendon (Levy), the composite longitudinal muscle (Morgan), or combined longitudinal muscle (Courtney), which encircles the rectum and the canal below the level of the levator fascia. It ends by splitting into numerous slips, the most im-

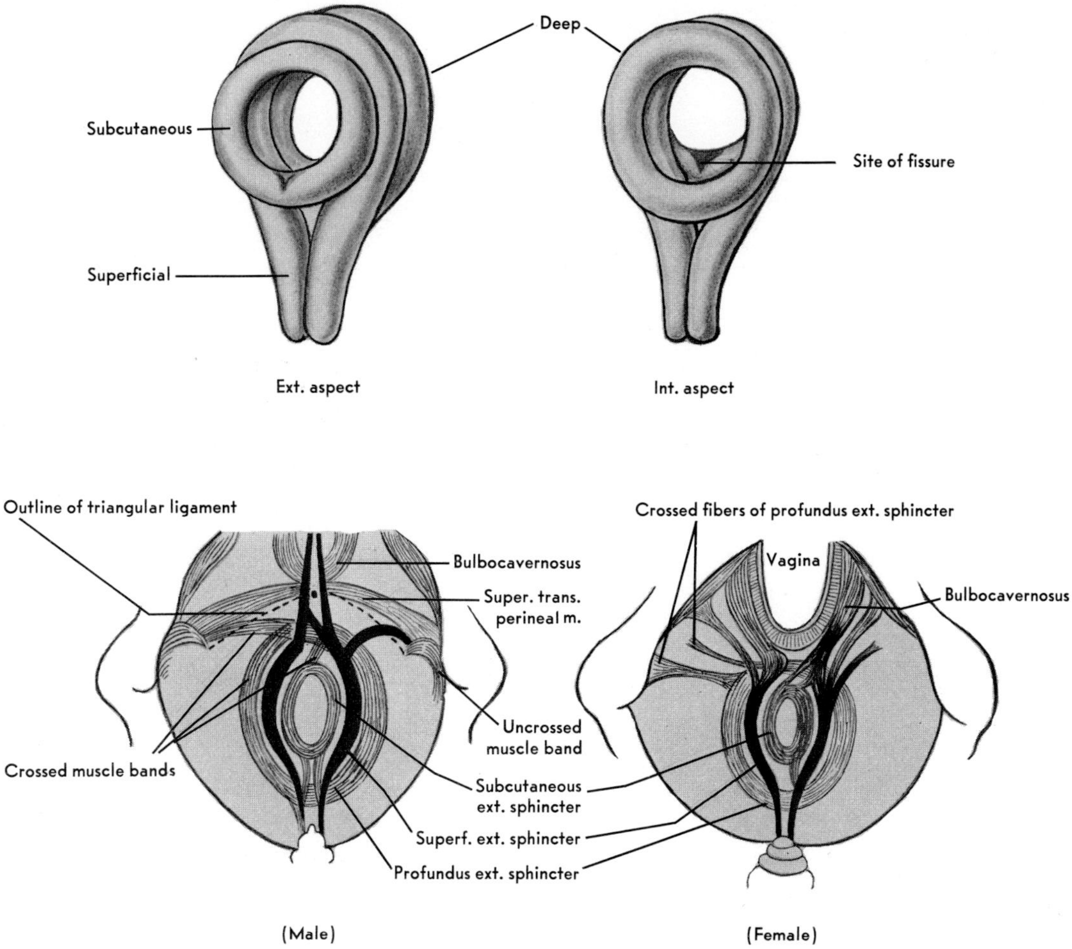

FIG. 32. Schematic drawing of external sphincter. (Redrawn from Gorsch)

portant of which are: (1) the anal intermuscular septum separating the lower border of the internal sphincter from the subcutaneous portion of the external sphincter; and (2) the perianal or transverse septum which separates the ischiorectal bands inserted to the perianal skin. The latter extensions are responsible for the formation of the normal radiating folds of the anus. This corrugator effect was at one time thought to be due to the action of a corrugator cutis ani muscle described by Elliot Smith.

The upper part of this longitudinal muscle band is in close relation to the ramifications of the preformed intermuscular anorectal fistula and the anorectal sphincter. At the lower part, the fibers may run medially to be inserted in the skin after penetrating the subcutaneous portion of the external sphincter and laterally to the subcutaneous tissue of the rectum.

The external anal sphincter is a voluntary muscle surrounding the lower two thirds of the anal canal. It is divided into 3 layers, as originally described by Santorini in 1715, by slips from the longitudinal muscle of the rectum.

1. *Subcutaneous portion:* annular, encircling the lower part of the anal canal, without bony attachment, and distinctly

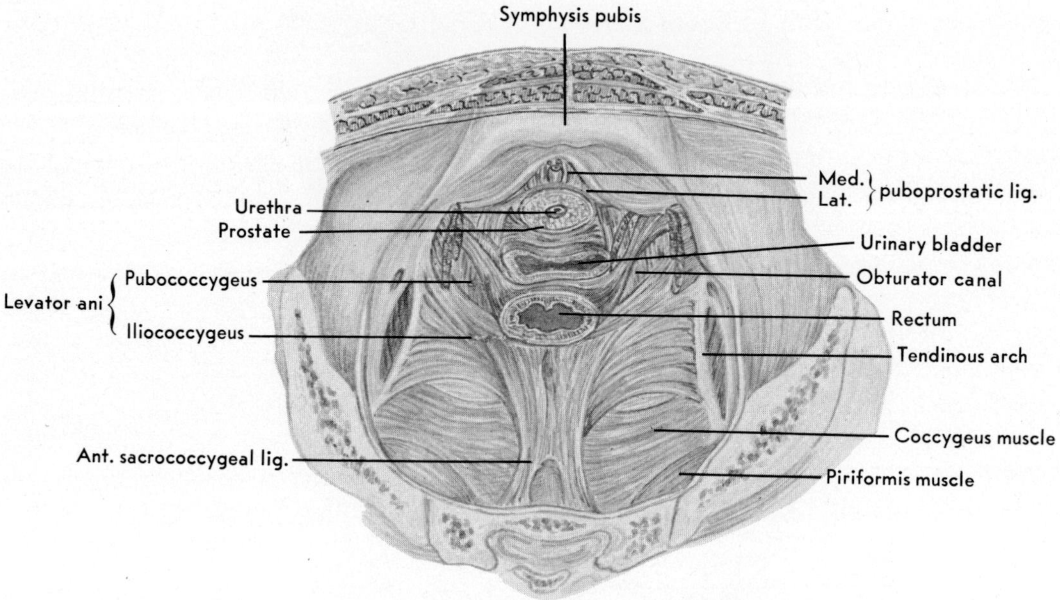

FIG. 33. The pelvic diaphragm (male).

palpable at the intersphincteric line. It lies below, a little lateral yet almost on the same plane as the internal sphincter from which it is separated by the anal intermuscular septum. Posteriorly, it merges with the fibers of the superficial portion of the external sphincter, while anteriorly it again joins extensions of the superficial portion of the external sphincter, together with the retractor scroti, the bulbocavernosus in the male and the sphincter vaginae in females.

2. *Superficial portion:* elliptical, consisting of 2 lateral halves which surround the internal sphincter, united anteriorly and posteriorly. Anteriorly, it is attached to the sphincter vaginae and the ischial tuberosities or the bulbocavernosus and the superficial transverse perinei muscles to the central tendinous raphe of the perineum. Posteriorly, it is attached to the anococcygeal body and through the anococcygeal raphe to the coccyx. It is into this muscle that a majority of the main tracts of anorectal fistulae open, and for a successful fistulectomy this muscle usually requires incision.

3. *Deep portion:* forms the upper third and is definitely palpable anteriorly, especially in females in whom it seems to be more prominent. It lies immediately above and slightly lateral to the superficial portion of the external sphincter. It is not attached to the coccyx and is associated with deeper fibers from the deep transverse perinei muscle. Anteriorly, the fibers decussate with those of the opposite side, and find attachment to the opposite ischial tuberosity. Posteriorly and laterally, the muscle is inseparably attached to the puborectalis portion of the levator ani.

The external anal sphincter usually is in a state of tonus, flattening and closing the anal canal. It is innervated by the inferior hemorrhoidal branch of the pudendal nerve (3rd and 4th sacral), supplied by branches of the inferior hemorrhoidal artery, and drained by the inferior hemorrhoidal vein.

While only a portion of the levator ani

seems to be directly related to the anorectal sphincter, it is probably best to describe the muscle as a whole. This fan-shaped muscle was described by Vesalius in 1515 and forms the bulk of the pelvic diaphragm. It was subdivided by Hall originally into 3 portions, later confirmed by Kolrausch, although recently Uhlenhuth stated that the muscle is really divided into 2 distinct layers, an inferior and a superior layer. It arises from the pelvic surface of both pubic bones and ischial spines, and the intervening white line attaches it to the pelvic fascia over the obturator internus muscle. It is divided by a distinct cleft into 2 distinct portions, with fibers of each portion differing in direction and depth of obliquity. These portions are the pubococcygeus and the iliococcygeus.

1. *Pubococcygeus,* more medial with the fibers running anteriorly, posteriorly directed backward and inward. It invests the urethra and the prostate gland; it is inserted into the lateral wall of the anal canal. It joins its fellow in the mid-line posteriorly, finally inserting into the anterior sacrococcygeal ligament. Anteriorly, the lateral halves are separated by the urogenital diaphragm. This portion is further subdivided by anatomists into 6 parts: (a) puboprostatic (pubovaginal in females) of which the fibers are related to and form a sling for the prostatic capsule (vaginal wall in females); (b) pubobulbar (pubourethralis in females) with fibers running toward the bulb of the urethra and to the bladder neck in males; (c) prerectal bundle of Uhlenhuth to the anterior rectal wall; (d) puboanal bundle of Uhlenhuth to the wall of the anus; (e) retrorectal bundle of Uhlenhuth to the posterior wall; and (f) puborectalis portion. Because of the importance of this portion, sometimes it is considered as a separate major part.

The puborectalis portion is essentially a U-shaped muscle, continuous on both sides, and lying a bit deeper than the rest of the levator. After passing around the lateral side of the vagina or the prostate and the rectum, it reunites with its fellow and forms an anorectal sling. It is a thickened roll of muscle, of which the axis twists at right angles after its origin with the result that the horizontal surface becomes vertical and the upper edge becomes medial, and the medial edge becomes inferior. When this muscle contracts, it increases the anorectal angle, drawing the anorectal junction close to the pubis and closing the anorectal lumen. It must be separated from the prostate in order to be able to liberate and mobilize the rectum. Medially, this muscle is intimately related to the longitudinal muscle of the rectum. Posteriorly, the fibers are inserted into the dense anococcygeal ligament and raphe.

2. *Iliococcygeus,* more lateral and becomes associated with the anorectal sphincters as they encircle the anal canal posteriorly. The iliococcygeus arises from the lateral pelvic wall behind the obturator canal, the ischial spine, with the fibers directed inward and downward to the side of the coccyx and the anococcygeal raphe in such a way that it is under a portion of the pubococcygeus muscle.

The levator ani muscle is supplied from the 2nd, the 3rd and the 4th sacral nerves through direct muscle branches from the plexus, and through the perineal branch of the inferior hemorrhoidal nerve arising from the pudendal nerve. This muscle serves in defecation and parturition and as a constrictor of the vagina.

The coccygeus muscle, called also the ischiococcygeus muscle, is the last of the original tail muscles. Posteriorly, it completes the middle part of the pelvic diaphragm. As a pair of triangular muscles spreading fan-wise it arises from the axial spine to the anterior surface of the last two sacral bodies and the upper coccygeal bodies. This muscle lends aid to the levator ani in supporting the abdominal organs and also helps to stabilize the sacro-iliac and the sacrococcygeal joints. It pulls the coccyx forward after defecation.

ANORECTAL RING

The so-called anorectal ring of Milligan and Morgan is a muscular ring that encircles the anal canal and the rectum. It is formed by the fusion of the internal sphincter, the puborectalis portion of the levator ani muscle, the combined longitudinal muscle of the rectum, and the superficial portion of the external anal sphincter. This anorectal ring is concerned with the preservation of the motor aspect of the anorectal ring which has to do with continence. Both the external and the internal sphincters may be cut, yet continence will remain if the longitudinal muscle bundle of the rectum and the puborectalis muscle are intact. The posterior attachment of these muscles to the coccyx prevents their retraction when sectioned. If the anorectal sphincters are cut in other portions, the cut ends retract, and the gap is filled by scar tissue, which impairs the efficiency of the sphincter control. The subcutaneous portion of the external sphincter may be cut with impunity, especially in operations for fissures, without any effect on continence.

Surgical Considerations

The anorectal sphincters are vulnerable to surgical errors in operations for anorectal fistulae. Unfamiliarity with the anatomy of the sphincters, lack of respect and improper technic may contribute to impairment of the defecatory mechanism postoperatively. This may be in the form of an annoying leakage to complete incontinence of feces. To prevent this complication, certain principles should be followed for division of the external sphincter ani muscles.

1. The muscle should be divided at right angles to the direction of its fibers.
2. The muscle must not be divided in two places at the same time.
3. Excessive retraction of severed muscle ends should be prevented by the insertion of one or more figure-of-eight sutures of chromic catgut.
4. Should it be necessary to divide completely all the components of the sphincter, this should be done in 2 stages by dividing first the deeper portions and surrounding the more superficial muscle bundles with a black silk seton tied loosely. Following firm healing of the deep muscle, the portion surrounded by the seton may safely be incised at a second procedure.
5. Packing inserted between severed muscle ends must be removed not later than 48 hours following operation and should not be reinserted.

ENDOPELVIC FASCIA

A discussion of the anatomy of the rectum and the anal canal should include reference to the endoabdominopelvic fascia. Under the peritoneum, one may visualize a continuous fascial sheath that lines both abdominal and pelvic cavities and invests the contained viscera, blood vessels and nerves and is intimately related to the underlying muscles and bones. Anteriorly and superiorly, it is continuous with the transversalis fascia; posteriorly, with the anterior layer of the lumbodorsal fascia and with the fascial investment of the iliacus and the psoas muscles. At the

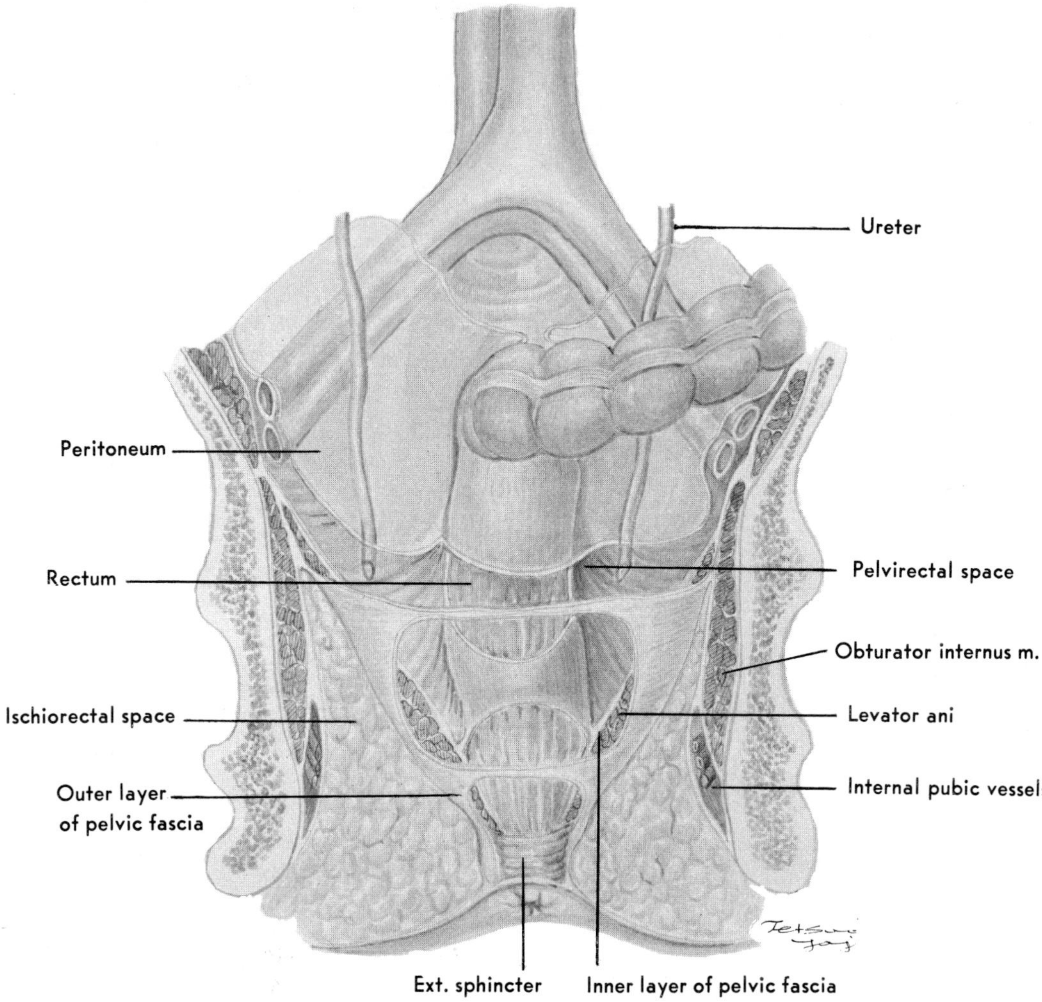

FIG. 34. The pelvic diaphragm and its fascia.

pelvic brim, the endoabdominal fascia merges with the endopelvic fascia. The latter is divided into 2 main parts: (1) an inner, dense membranous parietal layer that lines the muscles and bones forming the floor of the pelvic cavity, and (2) an outer, thinner connective-tissuelike visceral layer that covers the pelvic viscera.

The lateral and the posterolateral walls of the pelvic cavity are formed by the obturator internus and piriformis muscles as they overlie and smooth out the contour of the irregular pelvic bone. The sacral plexus and its branches course over the muscles and thus are invested by parietal layer, which is also called the ventral component of the hypogastric sheath. The fascial coverings of these muscles have been confusingly termed obturator and piriformis fascia, respectively; yet in reality they are portions of the parietal layer of the pelvic fascia. The blood vessels which are superficial to the fascia, unlike nerves, lie directly under the peritoneum separated by very fine areolar tissue. The posterior pelvic wall is formed by the

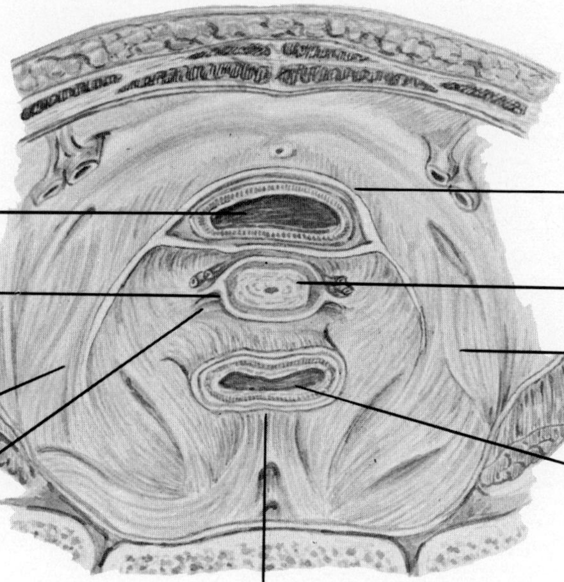

FIG. 35. The visceral part of the pelvic fascia (female).

sacrum with the sacral nerves emerging from its foramina. The sacral hollow is lined by a continuation of the parietal layer of this pelvic fascia. This is often referred to as the dorsal component of the hypogastric sheath. The floor of the pelvis is formed by the muscular pelvic diaphragm, which leaves a triangular defect in front, filled by the urogenital diaphragm just behind the pubis. All these structures are lined on the inside by the parietal layer of the pelvic fascia.

Resting on the pelvic floor are the rectum, the urinary bladder, the uterus and the adnexa. Their tubular conduits, the anal canal, the urethra and the vagina, respectively, pass through the floor. These organs are invested with the visceral layer of the endopelvic fascia.

The visceral layer of the endopelvic fascia extends horizontally across the pelvic cavity and is anchored or attached at its lateral edge to the parietal layer of the pelvic fascia along the linea terminalis which runs backward from the pubis to the ischial spine, close to the origin of the hypogastric arteries. This layer surrounds the urinary bladder completely, separating it from the vagina and the supravaginal cervix, and forms the base of the vesicouterine pouch. Then it passes up the body of the uterus to its peritoneal attachment; then it is continued posteriorly to cover the supravaginal cervix, the upper vagina, and the base of the rectouterine pouch. It finally surrounds the rectum, which it invests with a false capsule, and behind the rectum it blends with the presacral fascia, which is a part of the parietal layer.

The so-called Waldeyer's fascia is a stout avascular layer of parietal pelvic fascia that is adherent to the periosteum of the sacrum. It should not be stripped off but divided below the level of the sacrococcygeal articulation, owing to its intimate relation with the large thin-walled

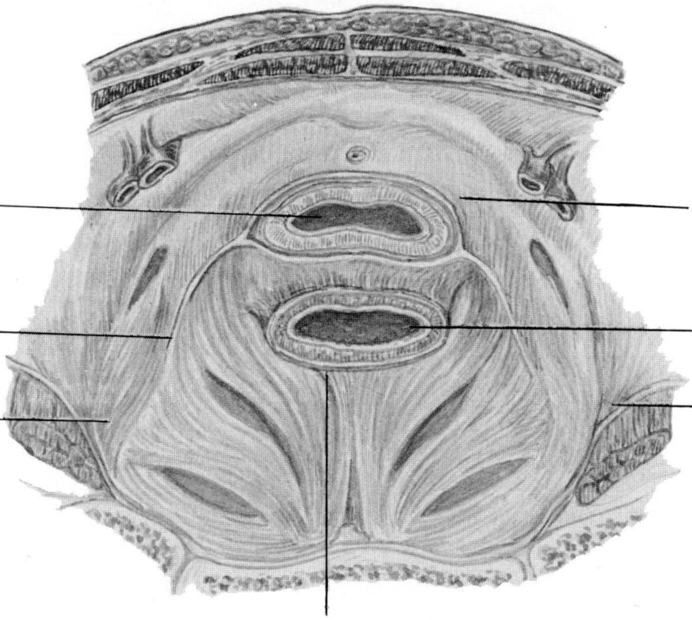

FIG. 36. The visceral part of the pelvic fascia (male).

pelvic veins, which macerate very easily and bleed profusely.

The so-called lateral ligaments or rectal stalks of Jonnesco are infoldings of the parietal layer of the pelvic fascia. They arise partly from the rectovesical fascia and with the areolar tissue about the middle hemorrhoidal vessels and nerves. All these structures form the middle hemorrhoidal neurovascular stalk.

In males, owing to the difference in pelvic viscera, the visceral layer has a somewhat different disposition. From the base of the bladder, the visceral layer is reflected upon the prostate gland, forming a false capsule of the latter. From here, there may be a rectovesical compartment which separates the urinary bladder from the rectum. Between the prostate and the rectum, from the pelvic peritoneum down to the superior surface of the pelvic diaphragm, is found Denonvilliers' prostatoperineal fascia or Tyrell's fascia. This fascia results from the fusion of the two layers of the rectoprostatoperineal fascia in the embryo. The anterior layer is adherent to the capsule of the prostate gland, especially at the junction of the ampulla and the ejaculatory ducts. The posterior layer is attached to the rectum. Between both layers is a potential space, the rectoprostatoperineal space of Denonvilliers or the rectoprostatic space of Proust, which is bounded below by the recto-urethralis muscle of Roux; the latter must first be cut to gain access to this space. A prerectal space between the rectum and Denonvilliers' fascia have been described by some and denied by others. Denonvilliers' fascia must be divided in order to separate the rectum from the prostate gland.

The visceral endopelvic fascia is more or less areolar in nature and not distinctly membranous like the parietal layer. The former is also called the pelvic cellular tissue and is not entirely confined to the

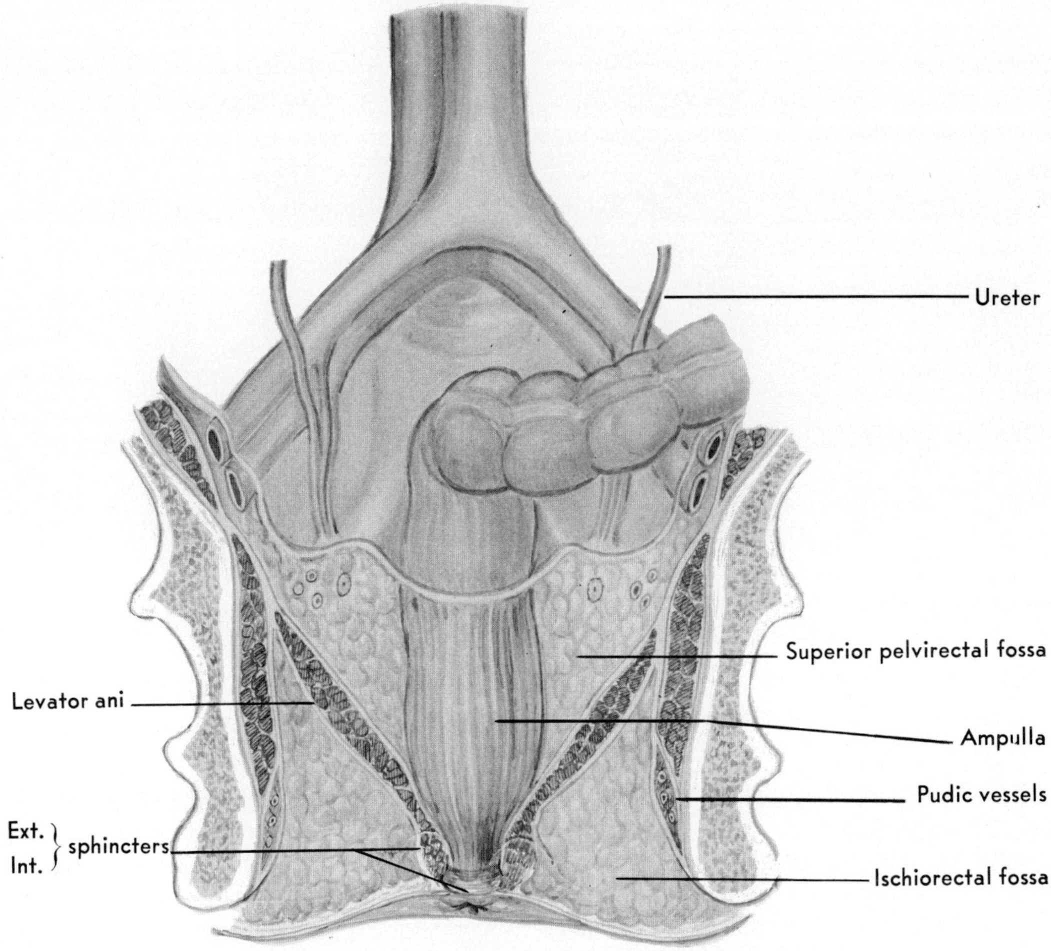

FIG. 37. Coronal section showing the pelvirectal spaces.

pelvis, being provided with numerous extrapelvic extensions. The latter pass through (1) sacrosciatic foramen to the obturator region of the gluteal area; (2) the obturator foramen to the obturator region of the hip; (3) the femoral canal to Scarpa's triangle; and (4) with the periurethral tissue to the perineum.

Certain fibrous condensations of the pelvic fascia, strengthened by the presence of smooth muscle and the areolar tissue intimately connected with nerves and vessels, have led to the formation of the false visceral ligaments like the cardinal ligament, the uterosacral ligament, and the round ligament of the uterus; the pubocervical ligament of the uterine cervix; and the subcervical ligament of the urinary bladder. Whether these ligaments can actually support these viscera is open to question.

PERINEOPELVIC SPACES

Numerous potential and actual spaces are formed in the perineum and the pelvis, owing to the presence of well-defined fibromuscular bundles and the contiguous fascial septa. The pelvic diaphragm with its contained levator ani muscle has been arbitrarily considered as the boundary between the two anatomic groups of spaces. These spaces are either above the levator (supralevator), below the levator (infralevator), and within the levator (levator) ani muscle plate.

Infralevator Spaces

1. **Perianal space of Milligan,** found in the lower third of the anal canal. It is bounded by the perianal skin below, the transverse perianal septum and the intermuscular septum from the conjoined longitudinal muscle bundle of the rectum above. It contains the terminal extensions of the conjoined longitudinal muscle of the rectum, the superficial perianal lymphatics, the external hemorrhoidal plexus, the inferior hemorrhoidal artery and nerve, and the subcutaneous portion of the external sphincter. The space is filled with firm, finely granular fat, which is more compact compared with the ischioanal fat.

2. **Submucous space,** found in the upper two thirds of the anal canal, between the anoderm and the internal sphincter and above the anal intermuscular septum. It is continuous with the submucous space of the rectum. It contains the inferior hemorrhoidal plexus with its supporting fibroelastic tissue and an extensive lymphatic network for the columns of Morgagni. A well-developed muscularis mucosa, called the sustentator tunicae of Kolrausch, has extension to the pecten of the anal canal, which together with fibers from the conjoined longitudinal muscle has been termed musculus submucosa ani of Fine and Lawes. When the intermuscular glands of Hermann are short, they only end in this space, and thus submucous abscesses could occur and even form fistulae without rupturing in the perianal area. When infected, owing to impaction of foreign bodies in the rectal lumen or due to the extension of inflammation from a fissure, a submucous fistula could also result.

3. **Postanal space,** found between the external anal sphincter and the coccygeal area. It is divided by the anococcygeal raphe into (1) a superficial compartment or posterior triangular space, the postanal space of Brick, which is actually the posterior part of the perianal space, extending from the intermuscular septum backward into the areolar tissue of the perianal region; and (2) a deep compartment which is bounded by the anococcygeal ligament below, the levator plate above, the external anal sphincter in front and the last two segments of the coccyx behind. This is also called the posterior communicating space or subsphincteric space of Courtney; it serves as a point where the two adjacent ischioanal spaces communicate.

4. **Subsphincteric space of Courtney,** found above the superior surface of the anococcygeal ligament which forms its floor, the decussating fibers of the deep portion of the external anal sphincter anteriorly, and the fascia over the last two segments of coccyx behind, and the inferior surface of the pelvic diaphragm above. This provides the posterior communicating space between the two adjacent ischioanal spaces and is actually the deep compartment of the postanal space. Actually, it is sublevator and retrosphincteric instead of subsphincteric.

5. **Postsphincteric space,** located between the anococcygeal raphe and the coccygeal attachments of the subcutaneous portion of the external anal sphincter. Its inner wall is formed by the pubococcygeus and the superficial portion of the external anal sphincter muscles.

6. **The para-anal or inferior pelvirec-**

tal space of Richet, actually a pair of spaces, each of which is bounded superiorly by the inferior surface of the pelvic diaphragm, inferiorly by the perineal skin, laterally by the pelvic wall and medially by the anal canal. This dead space allows expansion of the anal canal and the lower end of the rectum. This inferior pelvirectal space is subdivided by the segmental fascia or the lunate fascia of Smith into ischioanal and suprasegmental spaces. The lunate fascia of Elliot Smith is the fat-free deep fascia of the perianal region, whose reflection from the lateral pelvic wall is thought to form Alcock's canal, which contains the pudendal vessels and nerves.

A. ISCHIOANAL SPACE OR ISCHIORECTAL FOSSA is a roughly pyramidal or wedge-shaped fossa lined by infra-anal fascia and extending toward the urogenital diaphragm. It contains large locules of avascular fat, is incompletely traversed by fibrous septae. It lies below the lateral part of the pelvic diaphragm and measures 6 to 8 cm. in the anteroposterior diameter, 2 to 4 cm. wide, 6 to 8 cm. deep, and is approximately 60 cc. in volume. Its lateral or vertical wall is formed by the ischium, with the attached obturator internus muscle covered by the parietal portion of the endopelvic fascia called obturator fascia, and containing Alcock's canal. Its medial wall is oblique and is formed from above downward by the internal and the external sphincters, separating it from the anal canal, and posteromedially are found the perineal branch of the 4th sacral nerve. It is roofed by the segmental fascia, and posteriorly it is bounded by the gluteus maximus muscle where it is crossed by the perforating branches of the 2nd and the 3rd sacral nerves and the sacrotuberous ligament. Anteriorly, it is bounded by the superficial transverse perineal muscle and fascia. The two ischio-anal spaces are separated by the bulbo-anal and the sacrococcygeal raphes and communicate with each other through the posterior communicating space. In the male, the space is smaller, narrower and deeper, while in the female the boundaries anteriorly are not well defined. The ischio-anal space has two prolongations: (1) an anterior fossa of Waldeyer or pubic pouch, which is located between the obturator internus and the anterior part of the levator ani and the superficial fascia of the urogenital diaphragm, and (2) a posterolateral or gluteal pouch between the levator ani and the gluteus maximus muscle. The ischioanal space contains the inferior hemorrhoidal vessels and nerves, the posterior scrotal or labial branches of the superficial division of the perineal nerves, the deep branches of the perineal nerves, the perineal and the transverse perineal branches of the internal pudendal artery.

B. SUPRASEGMENTAL SPACES, a potential triangular space bounded inferiorly by the lunate or segmental fascia, laterally by the obturator internus muscle and fascia with Alcock's canal, medially from above downward by the inferior surface of the pelvic diaphragm and the upper end of the anal sphincters. It is free from fat and is easily demonstrable when filled with suppuration. Its apex is formed by the junction of the pelvic diaphragm as it is attached posteriorly to the ischial spine. At times, the levator ani is not attached along the linea terminalis, in which case an opening called the hiatus of Schwalbe is formed. It is through this hiatus that the pelvic peritoneum is pushed forward to form a hernia into the ischio-anal space. In other instances, the levator ani may be attached to the obturator fascia, only in several spots leaving multiple hiatuses through which purulent material may escape retroperitoneally.

An anterior communicating space between the two ischio-anal spaces is not generally recognized but it exists in relation to the superficial portion of the external anal sphincter. In the male, it is better identified because anteriorly the superficial portion may converge medially toward the central tendinous raphe, while in the female most fibers of the superficial portion of the external anal sphincter diverge laterally to the pubic ramus, fusing with the bulbocavernosus muscle.

7. **Posterior levator space of Courtney** is a wedge-shaped space found posterior and lateral to the rectum. When the levator ani nears the rectum, it divides into superior and inferior layers. Kolrausch and lately Uhlenhuth have pointed out that these layers are distinct and separate throughout. The superior layer is thinner and is more of an aponeurosis, while the inferior layer is thicker and muscular. As these layers diverge from one another, they leave a triangular space between themselves and the rectal wall. This is filled with loose areolar tissue and may become the site of an abscess. It is bounded medially by the combined longitudinal muscle of the rectum, above and behind by the iliorectococcygeus muscle (Courtney's term for the iliococcygeus and the rectococcygeus muscles combined), laterally by the superior fascia of the levator plate, and inferiorly by the anococcygeal raphe and the inferior fascia of the levator place.

8. **Perineal Compartments.** The superficial perineal compartment, while actually an infralevator space, is not of direct importance to the proctologist.

SUPRALEVATOR SPACES

A large subperitoneal area exists between the pelvic peritoneum superiorly and the superior fascia of the levator plate inferiorly, the pubis anteriorly, and the obturator muscle and fascia laterally, and the piriformis muscle and sacrum posteriorly. It is divided by numerous fascial wings extending from the different pelvic viscera.

These supralevator spaces are divided into an anterior urogenital and a posterior rectal compartment by the intervening fascial septum from the hypogastric sheath (the rectogenital or rectovaginal septum).

Anterior Urogenital Compartment

The division of the anterior urogenital compartment varies with the sex. In the female, it is divided into prevesical, retrovesical, rectovaginal and prerectal spaces. In the male, it is divided into prevesical, retrovesical and periprostatic spaces. The posterior compartment is divided into pararectal and retrorectal spaces.

1. **Prevesical or retropubic space of Retzius** is essentially the same in both sexes. It practically surrounds the urinary bladder and is divided into anteromedian and posterolateral recesses. The anteromedian recess is bounded by the anterior abdominal wall, from the level of the peritoneal reflection to the umbilicus above to the puboprostatic ligaments (pubourethral in females) below, and is in front of the urinary bladder. It is further subdivided by the inferior hypogastric arteries into a larger perivesical and a lower retropubic space proper. These lateral compartments are bounded by (1) the obturator muscle and fascia laterally, (2) the inferior hypogastric sheath medially, the endopelvic fascia inferiorly, as it gives rise to the ligament of the bladder, (3) the

superior hypogastric wing of the endopelvic fascia superiorly, and (4) the root of the hypogastric sheath and the ischial spine posteriorly.

2. **Retrovesical space** lies directly behind the urinary bladder and varies in disposition according to sex. Because of the interposition of the uterus and the vagina between the rectum and the urinary bladder in females, there is created the vesicouterine and the vesicovaginal spaces anteriorly and the rectouterine and the rectovaginal spaces posteriorly. In the female, the retrovesical or vesicouterovaginal space extends from the uterovesical peritoneal fold to the uterovaginal junction inferiorly; it is bounded (1) in front by the urinary bladder, (2) behind by the posterior wall of the cervix and the vagina, and (3) extends laterally to the uterovesical ligaments. It is divided by the supravaginal septum or vesicocervical ligament into a superior vesicocervical space and inferior vesicovaginal space.

In the male, the retrovesical space lies between the urinary bladder and the posterior surfaces of the seminal vesicles and the prostate gland anteriorly, the anterior wall of the infraperitoneal rectum posteriorly, the rectovesical peritoneal fold superiorly, and the superior layer of the pelvic diaphragm inferiorly. Into the middle of this space is thrust the rectogenital and rectovesical septum or the fascia of Denonvilliers or Tyrell, which can be further split into an anterior and a posterior layer with a space between them. Thus there are formed three spaces—an anterior retrovesical space proper between the urinary bladder and anterior layer of the fascia of Denonvilliers; a middle prostatic or the retroprostatic space of Proust between the anterior and the posterior layers of the fascia of Denonvilliers; and a posterior prerectal space between the posterior layer of Denonvilliers' fascia and the anterior rectal wall.

3. **Rectovaginal space,** bounded (1) anteriorly by the posterior vaginal wall, (2) posteriorly by the anterior rectal wall, (3) inferiorly by the fascia of the posterior vaginal wall and the anal canal at the perineal body, and (4) superiorly by the peritoneal fold of the rectouterine pouch. This is divided by the rectogenital septum into an anterior retrovaginal space and a posterior prerectal space. In the female, the rectogenital septum (counterpart of Denonvilliers' rectovesical septum) is not split into two layers.

4. **Periprostatic space** lies between the pubic bone anteromedially, the levator ani posterolaterally, the periprostatic fascia posteriorly. It is divided into a solitary anterior periprostatic space and a pair of lateral periprostatic spaces by the puboprostatic ligaments. The lateral periprostatic spaces are of interest because of the levator ani muscle, which forms its lateral boundary.

Posterior Compartment

The posterior compartment of the supralevator space extends on both sides and behind the rectum. It is bounded laterally by the pelvic wall and posteriorly by the sacrum. It has been divided into a pair of narrow pararectal spaces and a solitary retrorectal space by the intervening lateral ligaments.

1. **Pararectal space,** bounded by (1) the rectogenital septum anteriorly, (2) the hypogastric sheath anterolaterally, (3) the lateral ligaments posteriorly and (4) the rectum medially. In the female, this space is larger and is the most common site of abscesses in the supralevator space.

2. **Retrorectal space or presacral space**

is found between the level of the peritoneal reflection above, the upper surface of the levator ani muscle below, the sacral concavity with the presacral wing of the hypogastric sheath posteriorly, the rectum anteriorly, and the lateral ligaments anterolaterally. This space may connect with the other supralevator spaces, and these communications could explain the extension of retrorectal abscesses into the ischioanal space and other supralevator spaces and the sciatic notch. These spaces contain the branches of the sacral nerve plexus, the middle hemorrhoidal and sacral vessels. The nerves are found between the fascia and the muscular pelvic wall, while the vessels are found between the fascia and the subperitoneal areolar tissue.

Surgical Considerations

Of particular importance to the proctologist are the supralevator and the infralevator spaces when involved by infection and abscess formation. Anorectal abscesses are treated by immediate incision and drainage, except possibly the cutaneous variety. The opening of an anorectal abscess is governed by 3 rules that apply to the subcutaneous, ischiorectal (ischioanal), pelvirectal and retrorectal forms: (1) the incision should be in the anteroposterior direction or parallel with the anal slit; (2) the incision should be beyond the outermost fibers of the external sphincter but as near as possible to the point of maximum fluctuation; and (3) the incision should be of sufficient length to afford good drainage with excision of the skin edges in an effort to prevent premature closure.

Failure to open an abscess early may lead to extension of the suppurative process to adjacent tissues, following the point of least resistance and may result in a devastating effect on the anus and the rectum.

In subcutaneous and ischioanal abscesses, gentle attempt is made to locate the internal opening when possible, but one should not be too solicitous as to use force and create an artificial tract. Frequently, the tract will be found passing between the sphincters, with the internal opening located posteriorly in one of the crypts of Morgagni.

In the submucous variety of supralevator abscesses, incision and drainage are accomplished through the rectal mucosa. This may not require anesthesia, but if the abscess is situated near the anorectal line, some form of anesthesia is indicated. The incision should be made from above downward on the entire length of the abscess and along the longitudinal axis of the bowel. At no time should a transverse or cruciate incision be employed. The mucosal edges may be trimmed to prevent early closure of the cavity.

Pelvirectal and retrorectal abscesses are drained outside of the rectal wall and never through it. The incision is made on the posterolateral aspect of the anal aperture; with the guiding finger in the rectum, a closed hemostat is thrust in the direction of the abscess past the levator muscle, which is recognized by a sense of sudden "giving in." The hemostat is opened to separate the tissues for drainage. The skin edges are excised generously. One must be certain that the wound heals from within outward, and repeated probing may be necessary to accomplish this all-important aim.

ANAL PERINEUM

The perineum is a diamond-shaped space found at the inferior aspect of the trunk. It is bounded superiorly by the arcuate pubic ligaments, anterolaterally by the ischiopubic arch, posterolaterally by the sacrotuberous ligament, and inferiorly by the coccyx. An imaginary transverse line drawn between the anterior parts of the ischial tuberosities will subdivide the perineum into an anterior urogenital triangle and a posterior anal triangle. The urogenital triangle consists essentially of the perineal membrane and is not of primary import.

In the center of the anal triangle is the anal canal, which is bounded by the lateral para-anal spaces. Where the anal canal merges with the skin of the buttocks is the anal verge, or anal rim, or anocutaneous line. The anal opening is essentially an elliptical aperture disposed along the anteroposterior direction. Its edge is thrown into numerous radiating folds by the fibroelastic terminations of the conjoined longitudinal muscle of the rectum, the corrugator cutis ani, as it was once termed. The anus lies usually in the center of the anal triangle and is located in the mid-line just behind the intertubercular or interischial line. Bordering it and quite visible under the overlying perianal skin may be detected the rolled edge of the superficial portion of the external anal sphincter. The perianal region is lined by skin which contains hair, modified sweat glands and sebaceous glands. Occasionally, it may be darkly pigmented. Branched tubular glands belonging to the apocrine system are found surrounding the anal opening. These circumanal glands of Guy are responsible for the odor of the perineum. Being apocrine glands they are presumed to have some endocrinologic function, and their secretion differs chemically from that of the ordinary sweat glands. When infected, these glands form numerous intercommunicating abscesses which rupture, causing multiple perianal fistulae, none of which opens into the anal canal.

In the mid-line anteriorly, a prominent perianal raphe extends to join with the scrotal raphe, while posteriorly a smoother anal raphe leads to the coccyx.

The anococcygeal body of Symington consists of a mass of fibrotendinous slips extending from the anal canal to the tip and the sides of the coccyx and the lower part of the sacrum. It represents the fusion of the strong fascia of the glutei muscles, the levator ani, the superficial part of the external anal sphincter and the conjoined longitudinal muscle of the rectum. This separates the two ischioanal spaces from one another and divides the postanal space into a superior and an inferior compartment.

The coccygeal body (glomus coccygeum or coccygeal gland of Luschka) is a yellowish spherical mass 2 mm. in diameter. It is an aggregation of vascular nodules composed of arteriovenous anastomoses with nerve tissue and is probably of endocrine function. It lies anterior to the tip of the coccyx and is intimately related to the median sacral artery (which supplies it) and the sympathetic trunk. It lies within the anococcygeal ligament and below the levator ani muscles.

The rectococcygeus muscle of Treitz and Kolrausch (see preceding pages) is a triangular band of smooth muscle extending from the posterior taenia of the lower rectum to the pelvic surface of the 2nd and the 3rd segments of the coccyx. It is intimately related to the adjacent levator ani muscle and fascia.

The sacrococcygeal muscles are smaller ill-defined fibromuscular bundles that fill the space between the sacrospinous area and the last segment of the coccyx. It

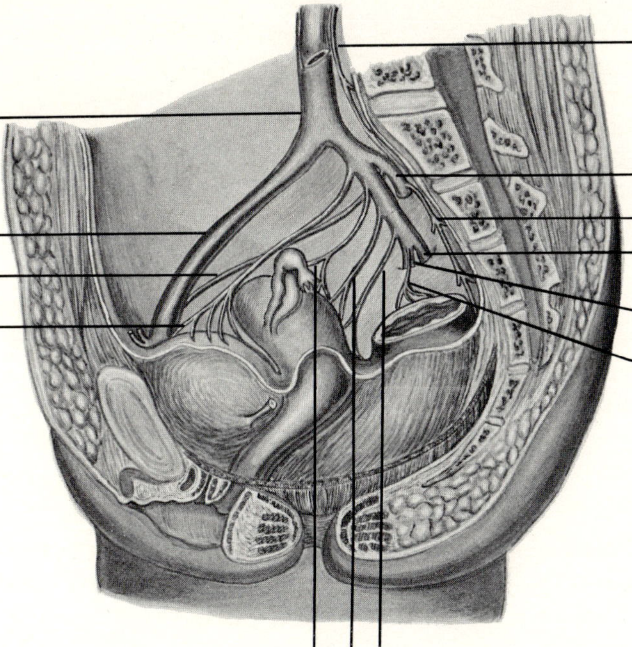

FIG. 38. Arterial blood supply of the pelvic viscera (female).

probably represents remnants of the vertebral tail muscles.

The central or fixed point of the perineum, while forming a portion of the anterior urogenital triangle, should also be familiar to the proctologist. It is a mass of fibromuscular tissue representing the condensation and the crisscrossing of the fibers of the external anal sphincter, the bulbocavernosus, the rectourethralis, the levator ani, the superficial and the deep transverse perineal muscles, and even part of the longitudinal muscle coat of the rectum. In men, it is located between the anal canal and the prostate gland and contains part of Buck's fascia, Colles' fascia and the superficial fascia of the urogenital diaphragm. In females the perineal body is a better-defined wedge-shaped mass of fibromuscular tissue receiving elements from the superficial and the deep transverse perineal muscles, the external anal sphincter, the levator ani and the bulbocavernosus muscles, together with loose areolar tissue between the anal canal and the posterior vaginal commissure. It has its apex directed toward the anus.

OTHER PELVIC STRUCTURES

There are certain pelvic structures which, while not part of the rectum and the anal canal, should be familiar to the surgeon.

PELVIC BLOOD VESSELS

The aorta usually bifurcates at the level of the 4th lumbar vertebra, a little to the left, into two common iliac arteries, each of which further subdivides into (1) a medial internal branch which supplies the

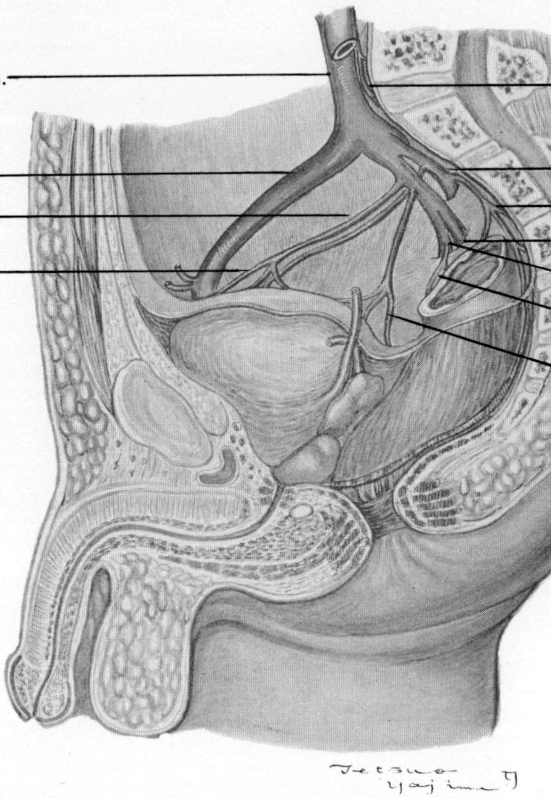

FIG. 39. Arterial blood supply of the pelvic viscera (male).

pelvis and the perineum, and (2) a lateral external branch which supplies the lower extremity.

The internal iliac or hypogastric artery has the following branches:

1. *Anterior division,* consisting of (a) 3 parietal branches—obturator, internal pudendal (which is the parent branch of the inferior hemorrhoidal), and inferior gluteal; (b) 6 visceral branches—umbilical, superior vesical (only in males), middle hemorrhoidal, uterine and vaginal.

2. *Posterior division,* consisting of only parietal branches—iliolumbar, lateral sacral and superior gluteal.

These arteries are accompanied by the corresponding veins. Purposeful ligation of any of these vessels may be done during the course of radical pelvic surgery. A rich anastomosis exists which ensures a good collateral circulation. Therefore, the internal iliac artery may be ligated almost with impunity. Localized engorgement with tortuosity of one or more groups of these vessels may occur in connection with the rapid growth and enlargement of pelvic tumors.

The pelvic veins have very thin walls and are very easily broken into. They lie beneath the peritoneum and, unlike the nerves, are not covered by the parietal pelvic fascia.

Ligation of the internal iliac artery has been our standard procedure in the excision of the rectum for the past 11 years. Here the collateral circulation is established by anastomosis between: (1) uterine arteries and the right and the left ovarian arteries; (2) vesical arteries and uterine and vaginal arteries; (3)

FIG. 40. The blood supply of the ureter: (A) male; (B) female.

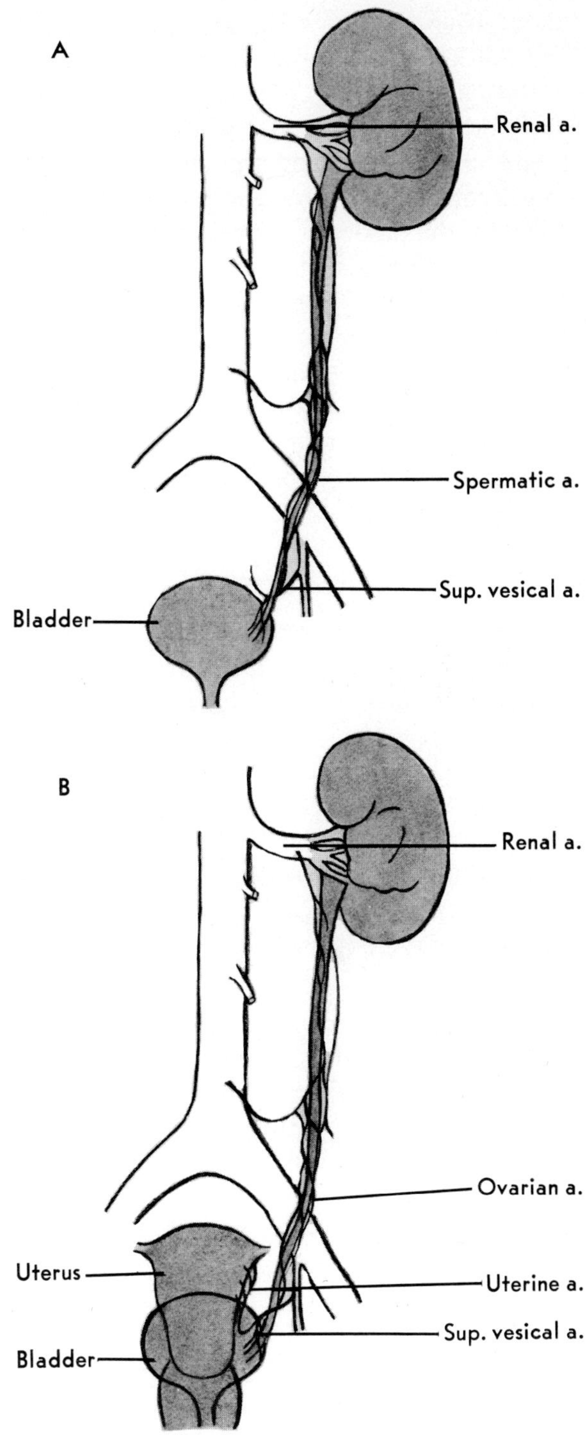

superior hemorrhoidal arteries and the inferior hemorrhoidal arteries; (4) obturator arteries and inferior epigastric arteries; (5) inferior gluteal arteries and circumflex and deep perforating branches of the deep femoral arteries; (6) superior gluteal arteries and lateral sacral arteries which in turn anastomose with the middle sacral artery; and (7) iliolumbar arteries and the lumbar branches from the aorta.

Batson's vertebral plexus of veins, a network of thin-walled valveless veins found at the front and the sides of the spinal cord, form a direct communication between the abdominopelvic veins and those of the axial skeleton and the brain. Normally, these vessels are closed, but retrograde flow occurs in them during increased intra-abdominal pressure. They have been blamed for the metastatic spread of pelvic tumors to the vertebrae and the brain without involving the liver and the lungs.

Pelvic Ureter

Another important structure with which one must be familiar is the ureter in its abdominal and pelvic portions. The abdominal part of the right ureter lies lateral to the inferior vena cava and is crossed by the right colic, the right gonadal (testicular or ovarian), the ileocolic and the superior mesenteric vessels. On the left side, the ureter lies lateral to the inferior mesenteric vein and is crossed by the ascending and the descending branches of the left colic, and left gonadal (testicular or ovarian) vessels. The ureter is very well drained by a rich intramural plexus of veins and is very richly supplied by an extensive periureteral anastomosis with branches from the aorta, and from renal, lumbar, gonadal (spermatic or ovarian), colic, vesical, middle hemorrhoidal, uterine, superior and inferior gluteal, obturator and hypogastric arteries. Corresponding veins drain into vesical, uterine, lumbar and renal veins.

In the male, the pelvic ureter crosses the external iliac artery, a point marked by the apex of the intersigmoid fossa of the left side, then runs along the lower border of the internal iliac artery to the ischial spine. It then runs forward and medially in the areolar tissue over the pelvic diaphragm, where it is crossed by the vas deferens overlapped by the seminal vesicles, and finally pierces the posterior wall of the urinary bladder obliquely, directed medially and downward. In its juxtavesical portion, it is closely related to the anterior rectal wall, and stones impacted in the former may be easily felt through the latter. The pararectal fascia is usually beneath the ureter as the latter enters the urinary bladder.

In the female, the pelvic ureter is closely related to the vessels and the ligaments of the uterus. It lies successively upon the uterosacral ligaments (where it is related to the uterine artery on its anterolateral surface), the cardinal and the vesicouterine ligaments (where it is crossed by the uterine artery) and as it enters into the urinary bladder it becomes related to the vesicovaginal plexus.

Surgical Considerations

In order to excise rationally all possible channels of lymphatic spread of carcinoma, more radical procedures and extension of lymphadenectomies have been devised and performed with improved results. When these operations are performed, there is that inherent danger of injury to important structures such as the ureters, the large blood vessels, the urinary bladder and the prostate in males and the vagina in females, which are in the immediate vicinity of the path of dissection. Therefore, a sincere effort to protect these structures at all times during the course of dissection is paramount to lessen postoperative complications in an already psychologically traumatized patient.

Ureters. The left ureter usually can be found at the apex of the intersigmoid fossa which lies on the left common iliac artery. The sigmoid colon is retracted medially to visualize the left ureter which not infrequently is intimately related to the inferior mesenteric vein, on the lateral side of the latter. Superiorly, the left ureter should be followed beyond the origin of the inferior mesenteric artery, and inferiorly along the pelvic wall where in its juxtavesical portion it is closely related to the anterior rectal wall. In the female the left ureter is closely related to the vessels and the ligaments of the uterus. While it is not possible to expose the ureter along its entire course its general direction may be obtained from the upper exposed portions. Care in the accurate application of clamps on bleeders deep in the pelvis can never be overemphasized, since lack of care is probably the factor that contributes most to injury of the ureter. The right ureter is better exposed at the pelvic brim. The same precautions should be observed, and particular attention is paid to this structure during clearing of the lymphatics related to the inferior vena cava, the aorta and its branches. As an added precaution, the authors make it a point to separate the ureters from the peritoneum to avoid its inclusion in the suture or possible kinking when peritonealization is carried out. Following these simple precautions, over 500 extended lymphadenectomies of the aortocavaliliopelvic groups have been per-

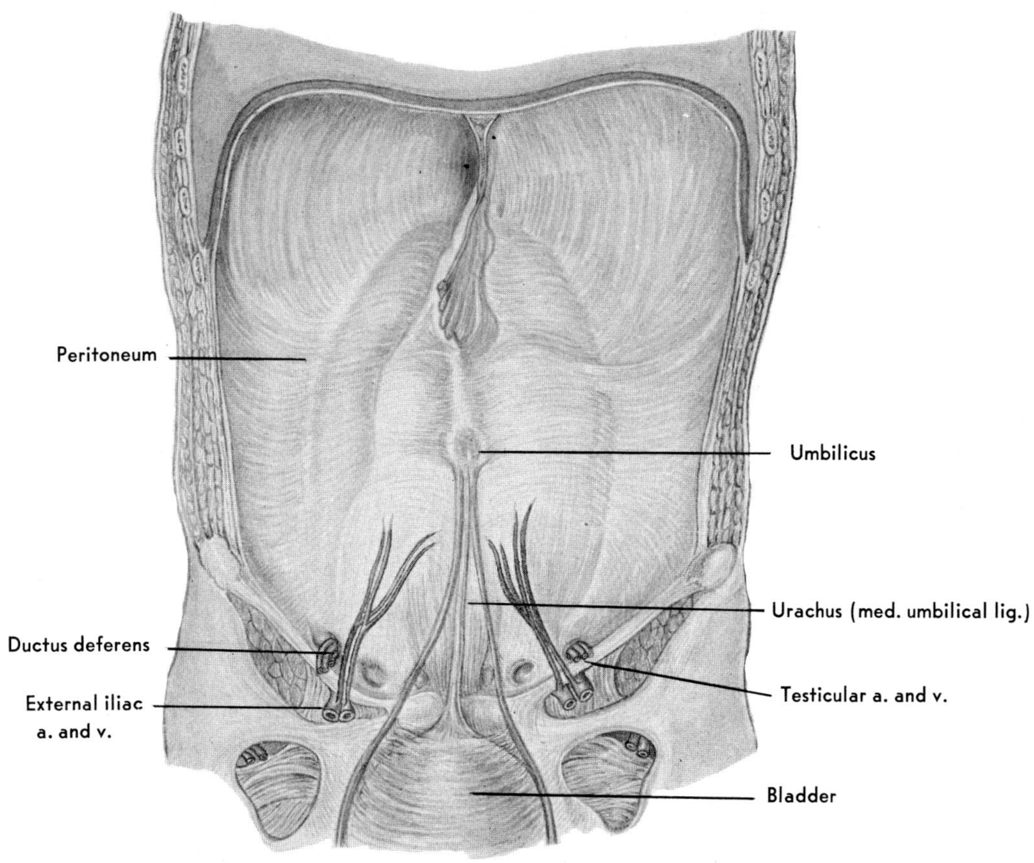

FIG. 41. Preabdominal peritoneum.

formed without a single instance of injury to the ureters.

Blood Vessels. Consequent to intense clearing of the lymphatic channels, the lymph nodes and the areolar tissue around blood vessels, troublesome bleeding is sometimes encountered, originating from the wall of arteries and veins. These are due to injury to the nutrient vessels and should be clamped accurately and tied.

A problem that is commonly encountered in operations for low-lying rectal carcinoma or carcinoma of the anal canal requiring a combined abdominoperineal excision (Miles') is the difficulty of providing hemostasis, which many a time has been the initiating factor for ligation of the ureter that has been included in a blindly applied clamp. To obtain hemostasis or keep the bleeding to a minimum, it has been the practice of the authors to ligate the internal iliac arteries prior to the pelvic dissection and perineal phase. The procedure is very simple, but utmost care should be exercised not to injure the underlying internal iliac vein which is thin-walled and can be easily traumatized. Therefore, the iliac vessels are exposed adequately and stripped of surrounding areolar and fatty tissue prior to ligation of the artery. Complications and increased morbidity have not been encountered following this procedure.

Urinary Bladder and Vagina. While these organs are intimately related to the anterior aspect of the rectum, injury to them could be prevented by carrying the dissection close to the rectum and in the proper fascial plane.

PERITONEUM

The surgeon must be familiar with the peritoneum. Like other serous membranes, the peritoneum is divisible into two distinct portions fused with one another along a line. The parietal portion lines the body cavity, while the visceral portion covers the contained organs with which it sometimes becomes inseparably fused as its serous coat. The reduplication of the visceral peritoneum upon itself, as it covers and supports the contained organ and is reflected back onto the parietal peritoneum, is called the mesentery of that organ. Thus the colon, or for that matter any organ, is never completely invested with peritoneum. There is always a small bare area posteriorly at its mesenteric attachments. The parietal peritoneum covering the anterior and the anterolateral abdominal walls and the undersurface of the diaphragm is comparatively smooth, continuous and plain, while that covering the posterior and the posterolateral aspects has an even surface depressed by several recesses of fossae, and its continuity is broken by the line of fusion with the visceral peritoneum.

The omentum is a duplication of the peritoneum which attaches the stomach to an adjoining organ. It is divided into a greater or gastrocolic omentum and a lesser or gastrohepatic omentum. The gastrocolic omentum is attached to the greater curvature of the stomach; it hangs down like an apron draped over and in front of the small bowel and, as it goes back to be duplicated upon itself, is fused with the transverse colon and its mesocolon. It is continuous with the gastrosplenic omentum on the left and the ascending colon on the right. Therefore, the greater omentum is composed of 2 descending and 2 ascending layers, all of which are derived from the peritoneum. There is a cavity between the 2nd and the 3rd layers, called the omental bursa or lesser peritoneal cavity, in the part above the transverse colon.

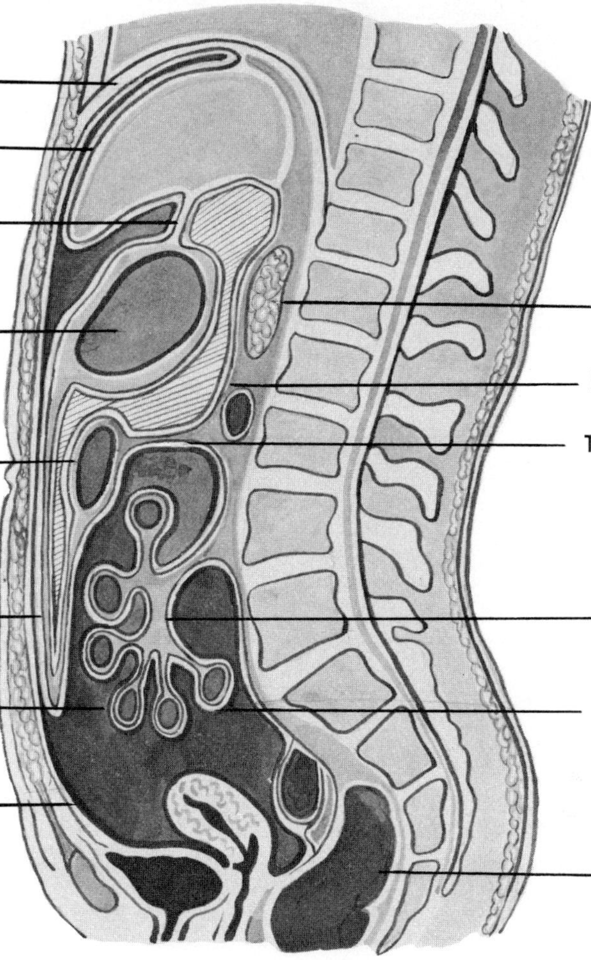

FIG. 42. Sagittal section showing the attachments of the stomach and the colon (relations of peritoneum and great omentum).

With the obliteration of the general omental cavity, between the 2nd and the 3rd layers, below the level of the transverse colon, and fusion of the 4 layers, the great omentum appears as a single compact structure with fat and vessels in its meshes. The attachment of the greater omentum to the transverse colon makes it appear as if the omentum takes origin from the transverse colon, along an avascular cleavage plane. The omentum is supplied by the left gastroepiploic branches of the splenic and the right gastroepiploic branches of the gastroduodenal artery arising from the hepatic artery. The omental veins drain into the portal circulation through the splenic vein.

The gastrosplenic or gastrolienal omentum connects the fundus of the stomach and the spleen. The gastrohepatic or lesser omentum arises from the lesser curvature of the stomach and the first portion of the duodenum and is attached to the transverse fissure of the liver.

The peritoneum has a free internal mesothelial surface and is mostly com-

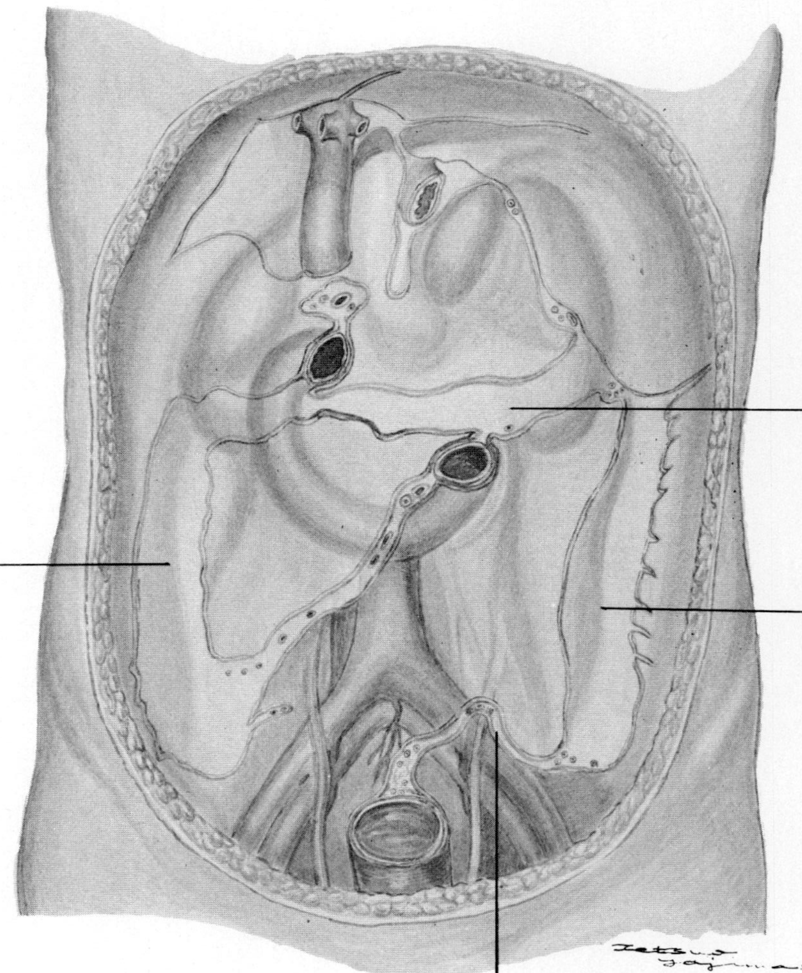

FIG. 43. Mesenteric reflections and usual areas of serous investment in the adult.

posed of fibroelastic tissue. The external surface is areolar tissue which attaches it to a viscus, the body wall, or to itself.

The cavity between the 2 layers of peritoneum is called the peritoneal cavity. In the male it forms a closed cavity, while in the female the abdominal ostia of the fallopian tubes connect the pelvic cavity to space outside the cavity. The peritoneal cavity contains only a minimum of thin fluid which allows the bowel loops to glide upon one another. The peritoneal cavity is divided into a smaller lesser peritoneal sac (omental bursa) and a larger peritoneal cavity related to most abdominal viscera. The two cavities are connected by the foramen of Winslow, which is bounded superiorly by the gallbladder, inferiorly by the superior margin of the first portion of the duodenum, anteriorly by the gastrohepatic ligament which contain the common duct, the portal vein and the hepatic artery, and posteriorly by the vena cava.

The general peritoneal cavity has an irregular posterior wall marked by numerous recesses. It may be divided roughly into two compartments by the interposition of the greater omentum and attachment of the latter to the transverse colon. The two compartments are the supra-omental and the infra-omental compartments. The latter is essentially the same as the inframesocolic compartment. The infra-omental compartment is divided into two roughly trapezoidal troughs, with a common central partition, the obliquely disposed mesenteric root. These are formed by (1) the transverse mesocolon above, (2) the attachment of the mesentery in the mid-line, (3) the pelvic mesocolon below and to the left and (4) the terminal ileum below and to the right. These are called the colic niches of Waldeyer or the colic triangles of Henke.

On each side of the vertical segments of the mesocolon is found a paracolic gutter or trough. The right half of the inframesocolic compartment is smaller and ends at the right iliac fossa, while the left half is larger and goes down into the pelvis.

Among the surgically significant posterior parietal landmarks related to the colon are the following:

1. Right renal pouch (Morris, Morrison) or the right subhepatic fossa of the supra-omental compartment of the general peritoneal cavity. The fossa is bounded (1) above by the visceral surface of the right lobe of the liver, (2) below by the mesocolic shelf and the anterior surface of the right kidney, (3) posteriorly by the epiploic foramen and the anterior surface of the lesser omentum. It communicates with the right paracolic gutter, which explains the spread of suppuration to the latter.

2. Left renal fossa of Hildebrand, analogous to the right renal pouch.

3 and 4. Right and left divisions of the infra-omental compartment of the general peritoneal cavity, the so-called colic triangles of Henke or the colic niches of Waldeyer. Through these spaces, the hepatic and the splenic flexures communicate with the pelvis below and the supra-omental compartment above.

5. Intersigmoid fossa or recess (de Haen, Treitz, Eve) which is found in 3 of every 4 bodies. It lies between the limbs of attachment of the pelvic mesocolon and is located where the psoas major muscle is covered by the pelvic mesocolon. It represents the incomplete agglutination of the primitive mesosigmoid and the posterior parietal wall. Its size varies from a mere dimple to an actual funneling several centimeters deep, with the apex di-

rected upward and to the left. In the case of an actual funneling, herniation into it can occur easily. A sigmoid artery lies above and to the right of it, while on its apex, the left ureter and the associated vessels cross the bifurcation of the common iliac artery. It is also related more medially to the superior hemorrhoidal artery.

6. Intermesocolic fossa of Broesike extends from either side of the duodenum to the edge of the attachment of the transverse mesocolon. It is covered by Broesike's intermesentericocolic fold extending from the transverse colon to the line of attachment of the mesojejunum. This contains the mesentericoparietal fold, which covers the superior mesenteric artery as it courses downward and to the right.

7. Duodenomesocolic fold on the left side lying over the left colic artery, and no corresponding fold on the right.

8, 9, 10 and 11. The 4 paracolic gutters are found on both medial and lateral sides of the vertical limbs of the colon, extending from the flexures to the pelvic cavity. Some authors would restrict the name paracolic gutters to the spaces lateral to these segments of the colon. These serve to channel inflammatory products from both the supra-omental and infra-omental compartments to the pelvis. At the base of each lateral paracolic gutter is found Moynihan's white line of physiologic fusion.

DUODENOJEJUNAL FOSSA

About the duodenojejunal junction are found several duodenojejunal fossae which may be the site of internal paraduodenal hernias. These are important, owing to the relationship that they bear to the superior and the inferior mesenteric arteries.

They are:

1. **Inferior duodenojejunal fossa,** directed upward, lying in front of the 3rd lumbar vertebra on the left of the ascending duodenum and is bordered by the origin of the inferior mesenteric vein. It is found in 3 out of every 4 bodies.

2. **Superior duodenojejunal fossa** is directed downward and lies in front of the 2nd lumbar vertebra behind the duodenojejunal fold at the duodenojejunal junction. Along its superior and lateral borders course the inferior mesenteric vein. This fossa is usually 2 cm. deep and is found in every 2nd body examined.

3. **Duodenojejunal fossa** which lies to the left of the duodenojejunal flexure, with its opening directed upward and to the right, usually is associated with some other duodenal fossa. It is usually found in 1 out of 5 bodies. Above it lies the duodenojejunal flexure and to the right the aorta, to the left the kidney; beneath it lies the renal veins; and anterior to it is the inferior mesenteric vein (which runs to the anterior wall of the fossa). An internal hernia into the fossa may compress the inferior mesenteric vein, slowing the return of the portal circulation and even resulting in the formation of hemorrhoids.

4. **Paraduodenal or inferior duodenal fossa** is bounded on the right by the ascending duodenum, on the left by a fold which contains the ascending branch of the left colic artery behind the aorta and in front by the duodenum. It is rarely present and may form a deep fossa extending behind the 3rd portion of the duodenum.

5. **Mesentericoparietal fossa of Waldeyer** lies behind the first part of the mesojejunum and is located on the right side with its orifice directed to the left. It lies against the 2nd and the 3rd lumbar vertebrae with the aorta a little to the left side. It is roofed by a peritoneal fold which contains the superior mesenteric artery.

Superiorly lies the duodenojejunal flexure. Small bowel loops can easily lodge here, but, owing to the wide mouth, strangulation is unusual.

MOYNIHAN'S LINE

The line of fusion between the parietal and the visceral layers of the peritoneum is indicated in the adult by a thickened, prominent, white streak called Moynihan's line of physiologic fusion. This marks the lateral edge of the avascular cleavage plane which permits relatively bloodless medial stripping of the related colonic segment from the body wall. This does not represent the actual point where the visceral peritoneum is reflected from the parietal peritoneum. It has been shown that prior to the agglutination there is an overlapping of the two layers. Later, the agglutination of these layers occurs by the contraction of fibrous adhesions which appear between them at the age of 7 to 9 months, and subsequently the intervening area of reduplication becomes absorbed completely. Thus the anterior longitudinal taenia are not facing anteriorly exactly but are turned a little to one side, because the colon is pulled laterally by the agglutinating layers. Occasionally, incomplete agglutination takes place, forming numerous parietocolic folds which produce intraperitoneal folds on the posterior body wall. Such areas as are incompletely fused prevent the medial spread of pathologic processes from the paracolic gutter to the retroperitoneal tissue.

ARTERIAL SUPPLY OF THE COLON

The colon is supplied by branches of both the superior and the inferior mesenteric arteries, which run between the leaves of the mesocolon and are distributed radially along its inner border, not unlike the ribs of a giant circular fan, making a diadromous arrangement. As these vessels approach the colon they usually divide into proximal and distal branches which anastomose among themselves, so that a more or less continuous fan-shaped vascular arch is formed all along, from the cecum to the pelvic colon. Occasionally, secondary and even tertiary vascular arcades may be found near the principal vessels. The vascular pattern of the colon is essentially the same, though less extensively as the small bowel. The presence of local disease, whether inflammatory or neoplastic, may make a certain portion of the vascular supply more prominent and tortuous.

The arteries of the colon are terminal in distribution, although minute submucosal terminal anastomoses have been described. These vessels then pierce the medial or mesocolic border perpendicular to the axis. The medial disposition of the blood supply is explained by the rotation and the transposition of the colon with the duodenojejunal flexure as its center. The absence of any major blood vessel of the colon allows one to cut the paracolic peritoneum almost with impunity.

Detailed and intricate anatomic description of the vascular pattern of the colon has been made time and again, but for practical purposes it is best to consider that every colon has its own original and individual vascular layout, and that while anomalies are not to be expected, their appearance should not be surprising. Adequate visualization of the vascular pattern, preferably by transillumination, should be made during surgery.

Superior Mesenteric Artery

The superior mesenteric artery supplies the derivatives of the midgut. It is around this vessel that rotation of the midgut occurs, with the result that those branches which originally run on the right side are found on the left in the definitive state.

The artery arises from the anterior surface of the aorta at the level of the 1st lumbar vertebra, 1 to 2 cm. below the celiac artery and usually is about the size of the common carotid artery. It may arise anywhere between the level of the lower third of the 12th thoracic vertebra to between the 2nd and the 3rd lumbar vertebrae, although usually it arises between the 1st and the 2nd lumbar vertebrae. In 1 per cent of bodies it may arise in common with the celiac artery.

The prearterial segment of the midgut, i.e., the portion from the duodenum to the ileocecal area, has its branches arising from the convex border, while the postarterial segment, i.e., from the cecoappendiceal region to the midtransverse colon, has its branches arising from the right concave border.

After arising from the aorta, it passes beneath the pancreas, between the head and the neck of the organ; then below its

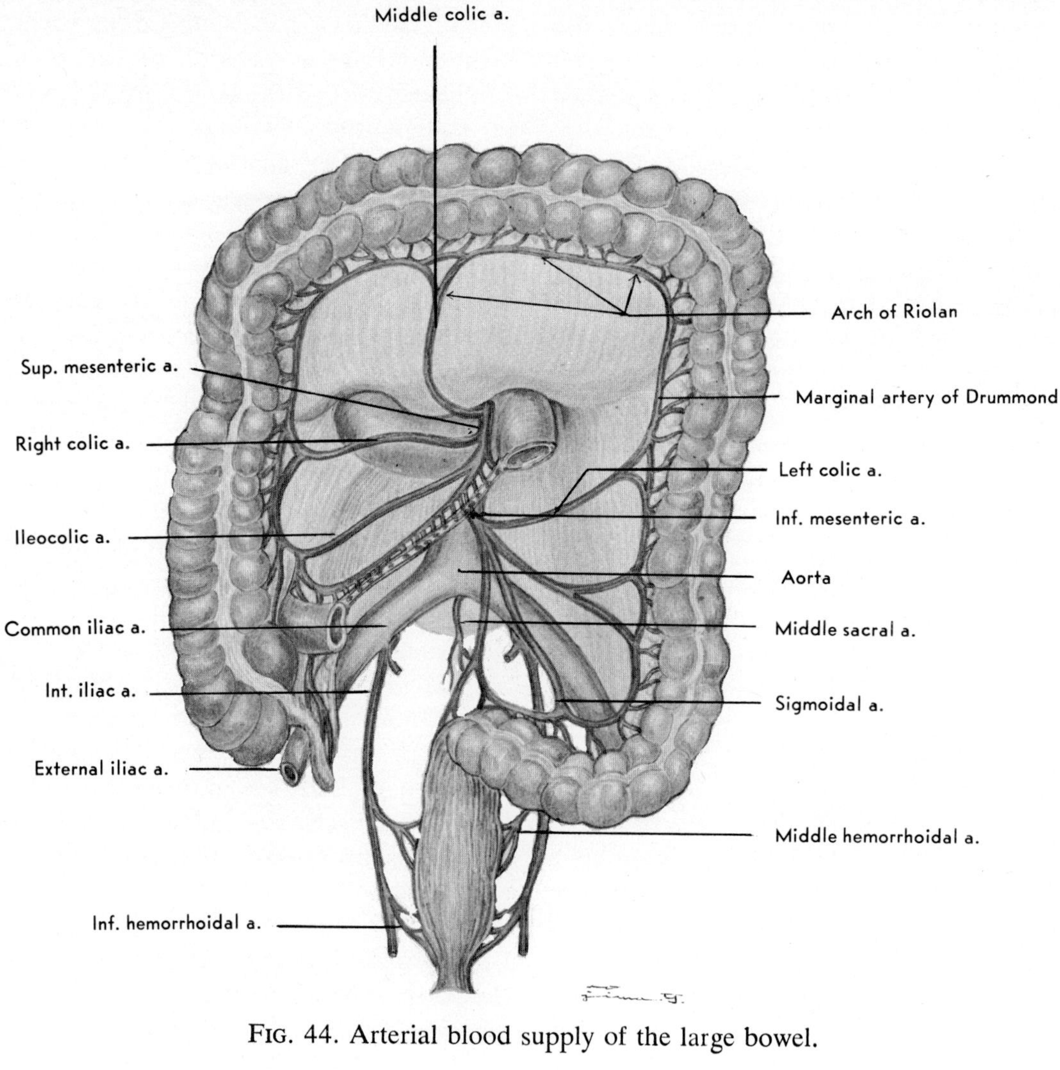

FIG. 44. Arterial blood supply of the large bowel.

border it crosses the third part of the duodenum before entering the mesentery proper.

Between the leaves of the mesentery, the artery passes downward to the right iliac fossa, where it ends by forming an anastomotic vascular arcade with one of its own branches, the ileal branch of the ileocolic artery. At its origin it lies behind the splenic vein and the pancreas, where it is also crossed by the transverse mesocolon in front. Behind it lies the left renal vein. As it enters the mesenteric root, it crosses the third part of the duodenum, the aorta, the inferior vena cava, the right ureter, the right gonadal (testicular or ovarian) vessels and the right psoas major muscle. Around it are the sympathetic fibers from the celiac plexus that form the superior mesenteric plexus. The accompanying superior mesenteric vein lies to its right side, either in front or behind the ileocolic artery or the right colic artery.

Branches of the Superior Mesenteric Artery:

1. *Inferior pancreaticoduodenal,* which is given off close to the origin of the superior mesenteric artery as it emerges under the pancreas, and is the only branch that arises from the right side yet does not supply the large bowel. The branches of the inferior pancreaticoduodenal, together with the branches of the superior pancreaticoduodenal, form the anterior and the posterior vascular arcades on the head of the pancreas.

2. A dozen or more *jejunal and ileal branches* arising and spreading radially from the left convex border, forming vascular arcades between the leaves of the mesentery, the short terminal branches of which are finally distributed to the jejunum and the ileum.

3. *Middle colic artery* is the first colic branch of the superior mesenteric artery and arises from the right concave side about 1 cm. below the inferior pancreaticoduodenal artery and therefore below the pancreas. The artery enter the transverse mesocolon and thus lies behind the stomach, passing downward, forward and to the right. It is called the middle colic because it supplies the middle or transverse segment of the colon and not because it is supposed to lie in the mid-line. Drawing the greater omentum and reflecting the transverse mesocolon upward would show the middle colic artery crossing to the right. To its left would be the wide avascular area of Riolan, which is the ideal and convenient space to go through the transverse mesocolon in order to gain access to the posterior wall of the stomach when performing a posterior gastrojejunal anastomosis. Since the middle colic lies in the transverse mesocolon, it is situated behind the stomach, and, owing to the fusion of the floor of the omental bursa and the transverse mesocolon, the middle colic may be easily ligated inadvertently when the gastroepiploic vessels are tied while liberating the stomach prior to gastroectomy.

The middle colic artery divides into (a) the right branch, which supplies the proximal or right third of the transverse colon and anastomoses with the ascending or superior branch of the right colic artery near the hepatic flexure; (b) the left branch, which supplies the left or distal two thirds of the transverse colon and anastomoses with the ascending or superior branch of the left colic artery.

4. *Right colic,* which arises 1 to 3 cm. below the middle colic and passes to the right behind the peritoneum a little below the inferior pole of the right kidney, run-

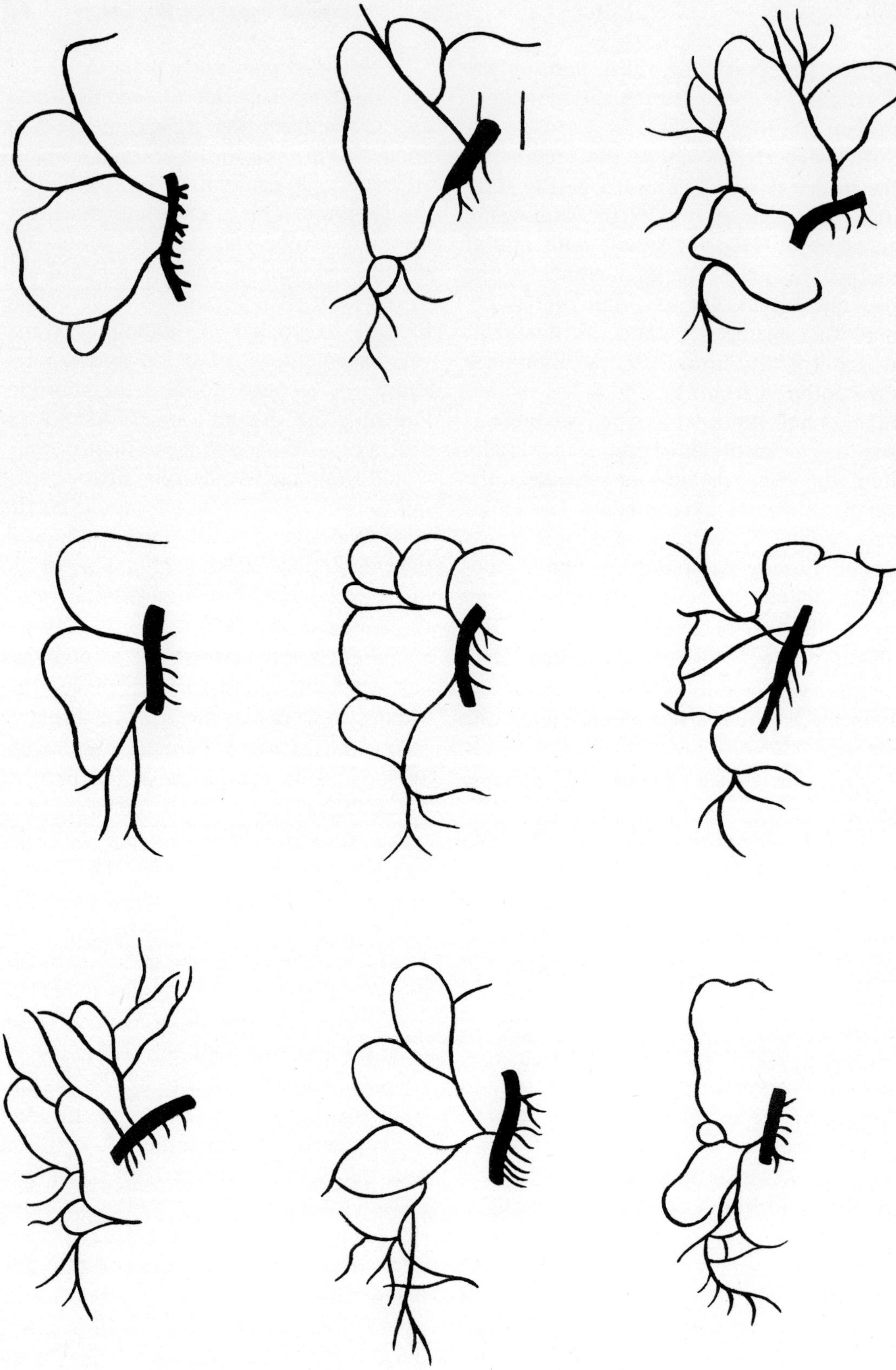

ning in the posterior wall of the right inframesocolic compartment. It crosses in front of the inferior vena cava, the right psoas major muscle, the right gonadal (testicular or ovarian) vessels and the right ureter. At the level of the midascending colon it usually divides into (a) ascending or distal branches, which pass upward and anastomose with the right branch of the middle colic in the transverse mesocolon, and (b) descending or proximal branches, which pass downward and anastomose with the ascending branch of the ileocolic artery.

5. *Ileocolic artery,* a constant terminal branch of the superior mesenteric artery that supplies the terminal ileum, the ceco-appendiceal region and the proximal ascending colon. It arises opposite the upper jejuno-ileal arteries and descends to the right toward the ileocecal valve. Its branches vary in origin and size. Its terminal branches are: (a) ascending or superior branches which anastomose with the descending or proximal branches of the right colic; (b) descending or inferior branches which divide into anterior and posterior cecal arteries (that supply the corresponding walls of the cecum), appendicular (appendiceal artery in the mesoappendix, that goes to supply the vermiform appendix), ileal (to the terminal ileum), and anastomose with the ileal branches of the superior mesenteric artery.

Variations. There are a number of variations from the above standard arborization of the arterial supply of the colon.

1. *The middle colic and the right colic arteries* arise as a common trunk from the superior mesenteric artery in about 6 of 20 bodies. In these cases there are only two arteries that supply both hemicolon: a right hemicolic and a left colic artery. The ileocolic artery in such instances may arise as a separate trunk.

2. *The right colic* is totally absent in 4 out of 20 bodies, although in only 8 out of 20 bodies is it derived from the superior mesenteric artery. Its place is taken by large secondary descending colic branches from the middle colic and the ascending colic branches from the ileocolic artery.

3. *The right colic and ileocolic arteries* have a common trunk in 2 out of 20 bodies.

4. *The middle colic* is absent in 1 out of 20 bodies. In such cases a large right colic artery with large ascending branches may take its place.

5. *An accessory middle colic* arises from the superior mesenteric artery in 2 out of 20 bodies.

6. *An accessory right colic* may arise from either the right colic or the middle colic artery.

7. *The right colic* may give rise to an accessory right colic or ileocolic arteries, which is functionally identical as a single common trunk for the right colic and the ileocolic. Ligature of the superior mesenteric artery or thrombosis or embolism of this vessel results in hemorrhagic infarction.

Inferior Mesenteric Artery

The inferior mesenteric artery supplies the left hemicolon and the proximal part of the rectum. It is almost always present, having been reported in only one instance, in which there was a double superior

FIG. 45. Colic and cecal arteries. Variations encountered in 200 specimens. The patterns are arranged in the order of decreasing frequency. (Redrawn from Sonneland and Anson)

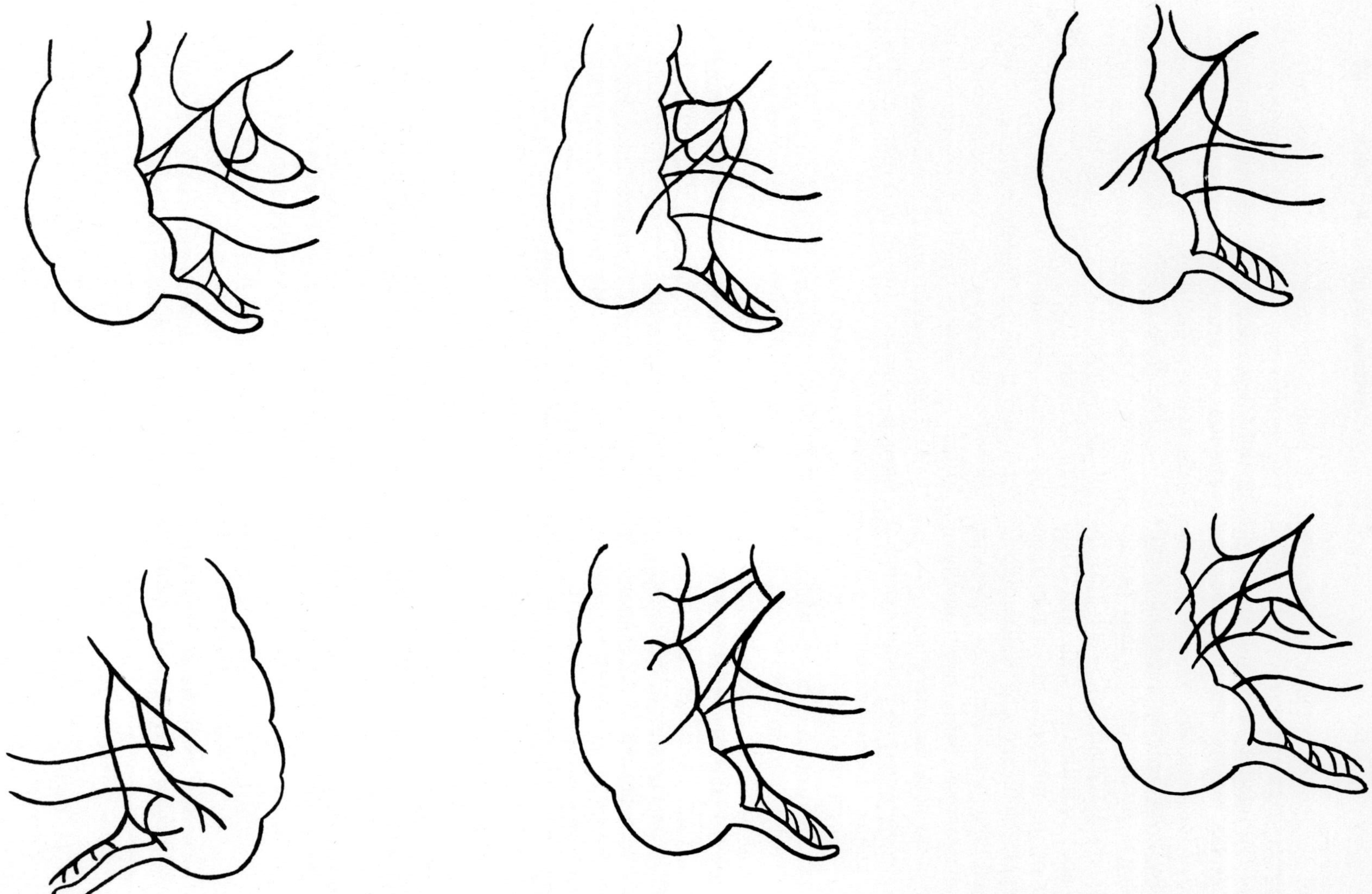

FIG. 46. Appendiceal and cecal arteries: major variations encountered in 200 specimens. (Redrawn from Beaton, Anson)

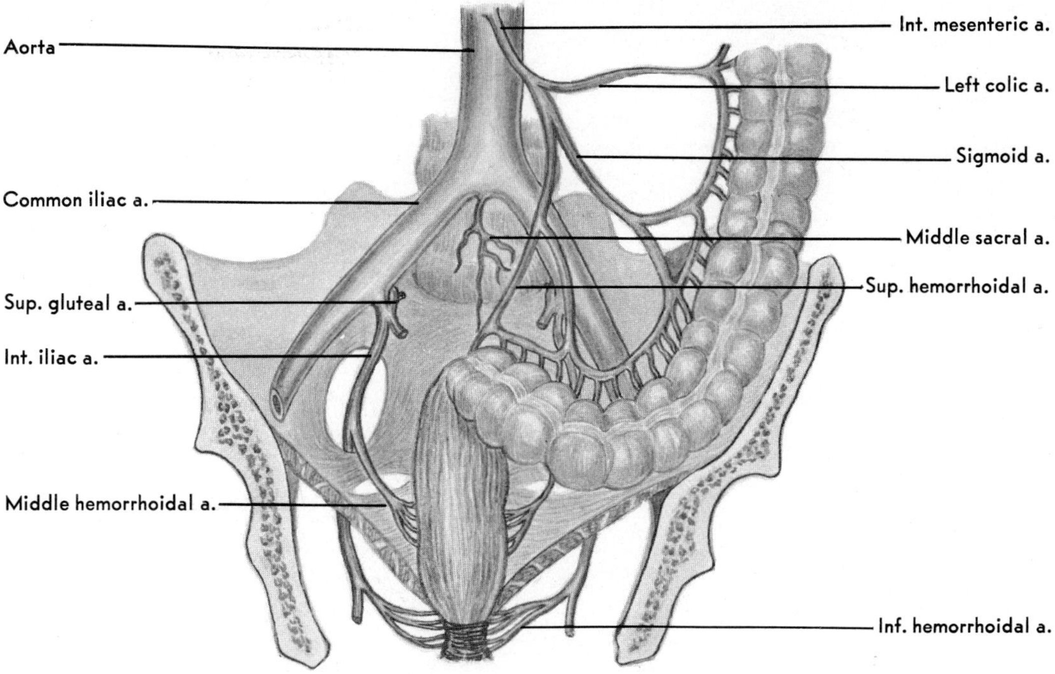

FIG. 47. Arterial blood supply of the sigmoid and the rectum.

mesenteric artery and no inferior mesenteric artery. The artery arises from the anterior surface of the aorta at a variable distance from the aortic bifurcation. In general, it arises 5 to 6 cm. above the bifurcation, with a range of 3 to 9 cm. It may even be located above the lowest portion of the duodenal curve, in which case the duodenum must be reflected away from the body wall in order to ligate the inferior mesenteric artery at its origin. It may be found from the level of the lower half of the 2nd lumbar vertebra to the upper half of the 4th lumbar vertebra, although it is often found at the level of the 3rd lumbar vertebra. It then courses downward over the psoas major muscle, entering the base of the mesosigmoid, then crosses the left common iliac artery and becomes the superior hemorrhoidal or superior rectal artery as it enters the pelvis. The inferior mesenteric artery is smaller than the superior mesenteric and is of more constant and limited distribution. It is surrounded by sympathetic fibers derived from the aortic plexus. Its accompanying vein lies about 2 cm. lateral from it.

Branches of the inferior mesenteric:

1. *Left colic artery,* which arises from the left side of the inferior mesenteric artery below the duodenum, usually within 2 to 4 cm. of the aortic origin of the latter. It passes subperitoneally to the left and crosses the left gonadal (testicular or ovarian) vessels and the left ureter and the inferior mesenteric veins at a variable distance. It divides into: (a) an ascending branch that crosses the lower pole of the left kidney as it runs upward and to the left toward the splenic flexure and divides into a branch that anastomoses with the left branch of the middle colic, and a branch that supplies the upper half of the descending colon; (b) a descending branch that passes to the left and

divides into ascending branches which anastomose with the descending colic branch of the ascending branch of the left colic, and descending colic branches that supply the lower half of the descending colon.

2. *Sigmoid artery,* that is usually a single trunk called the inferior left colic artery. It further subdivides into at least a pair of arteries, occasionally as many as 4. These arteries pass downward to the left toward the iliac portion of the descending colon, lie behind the peritoneum and cross the left psoas major muscle, the left ureter, the left iliacus muscle and the left gonadal (testicular or ovarian) vessels. The sigmoid artery divides into branches that anastomose with the left colic artery and the superior hemorrhoidal artery; it supplies the descending and the pelvic portions of the colon. In some instances each sigmoidal artery may arise as a separate trunk from the inferior mesenteric artery.

The lowermost sigmoidal artery may not anastomose with the superior hemorrhoidal artery, or it may have a narrow frail communicating trunk—the rectosigmoid artery of Pope. Because of this apparently weak spot, it has been previously advised that ligation of the superior hemorrhoidal artery be accomplished above the lowermost sigmoid, if viability of the bowel is not to be compromised. This is called the critical point of Sudeck or Hartmann, and this teaching or belief retarded the early progress of surgery of the rectosigmoidal region for a number of years. Clinical experience has proved that the superior hemorrhoidal artery may be ligated anywhere without compromising viability of the rectum and the rectosigmoid. This is accounted for by the so-called marginal artery of Drummond, and probably the extensive collateral circulation from the middle and the inferior hemorrhoidal arteries, that can supply the rectum from below.

3. *Superior hemorrhoidal* or superior rectal artery, that is the continuation of the inferior mesenteric artery which runs in the mesosigmoid and crosses the left common iliac artery, then proceeds toward the median line, where behind the rectosigmoid junction it divides into two terminal branches which descend on each side of the rectum.

Marginal Artery

Von Haller had noted long ago the continuous vascular arcade referred to as Drummond's marginal artery. This makes possible the continuity of the vascular channel from the cecum down to the sigmoid colon, even if the major colic arteries are ligated at their origins. Archibald has previously shown, and our operative experience has borne out the fact, that the marginal artery when intact can maintain the blood supply of the colon even if the inferior mesenteric artery is ligated at the point of origin from the aorta. The rich anastomoses, whether by single connecting trunks or by vascular arcades (primary, secondary and tertiary), which abound near the flexures, form essentially a single arterial trunk from the terminal ileum to the sigmoid colon. This arterial trunk may lie anywhere from one to several centimeters from the mesocolic margin of the bowel and is thus referred to as the marginal artery. In the more movable segments of the colon, the marginal vascular arch is generally farther away from the bowel.

Riolan noted a large anastomotic vessel that connects the middle and the left colic arteries in the transverse mesocolon. Essentially, this vessel represents a communication between the superior and the inferior mesenteric arteries.

The terminal distribution of the marginal artery to the large bowel follows a more or less regular pattern, which has been studied extensively by Rankin. The marginal artery in the mesocolon gives off parallel closely spaced sets of 3 branches which are distributed for short distances only to limited segments of the bowel wall. A pair of long branches—one anterior and another posterior—pierce the bowel wall between the mesocolic and the lateral taenia to pass around the front and the back of the gut, respectively. They course between the serous and the muscular coats of the colon until they almost reach the medial taenia which is amesocolic, away from the mesocolon on the opposite side. At this point they penetrate the muscular coat to ramify in the submucosa, in which the anterior and the posterior branches may effect a minimal terminal anastomosis, midway between the two mesocolic taenia. On the other hand, the solitary short terminal branch, which may arise direct from the marginal artery or from either of the long branches, penetrates immediately into the submucosa without branching, at the region of the mesocolic or the posteromedial taenia. The base of the appendices epiploicae is usually related to the circularly disposed vessels, particularly the short branches of the marginal artery which courses near the base. It is imperative that when the appendix epiploica is to be cut, it should not be cut flush with the bowel wall. Further, in cutting, no traction should be made on the fat tab in order to prevent injury to these short branches. The site of the appendices epiploicae and the point where the vessels pierce the wall obliquely represent points of mural weakness; thus, diverticulae may arise in relation to them at these points. Diverticulitis is essentially identical with inflammation of the epiploic appendage that contains the inflamed diverticulum. The relation of the central arterial core to the venous coil about it in the appendix epiploica is also a factor in the pathogenesis of torsion of the appendices epiploicae.

Thus the mesenteric part of the colon is better supplied with blood. Consequently, in performing anastomosis it is wise to sacrifice a greater part of the amesocolic area, with an obliquely disposed cut, in order to ensure viability of the wound edge and also a wider lumen.

ARTERIAL SUPPLY OF THE RECTUM AND THE ANAL CANAL

The rectum and the anal canal are supplied by 3 pairs of hemorrhoidal or rectal arteries (superior, middle and inferior) and the middle sacral artery.

Superior Hemorrhoidal Artery

The superior hemorrhoidal artery originates as the direct continuation of the inferior mesenteric artery at the upper and outer border of the left common iliac artery. It descends into the pelvis in the root of the mesosigmoid, coursing toward the median line, in the superior hemorrhoidal neurovascular sheath of the rectum. Behind the rectosigmoid, while still in the mesorectum, it bifurcates into right and left branches. This level of bifurcation varies with the height of the rectum. These main branches pierce the muscular coat and then descend under cover of the lateral peritoneal reflection along the posterolateral aspect of the rectum. It supplies the whole mural surface of the rec-

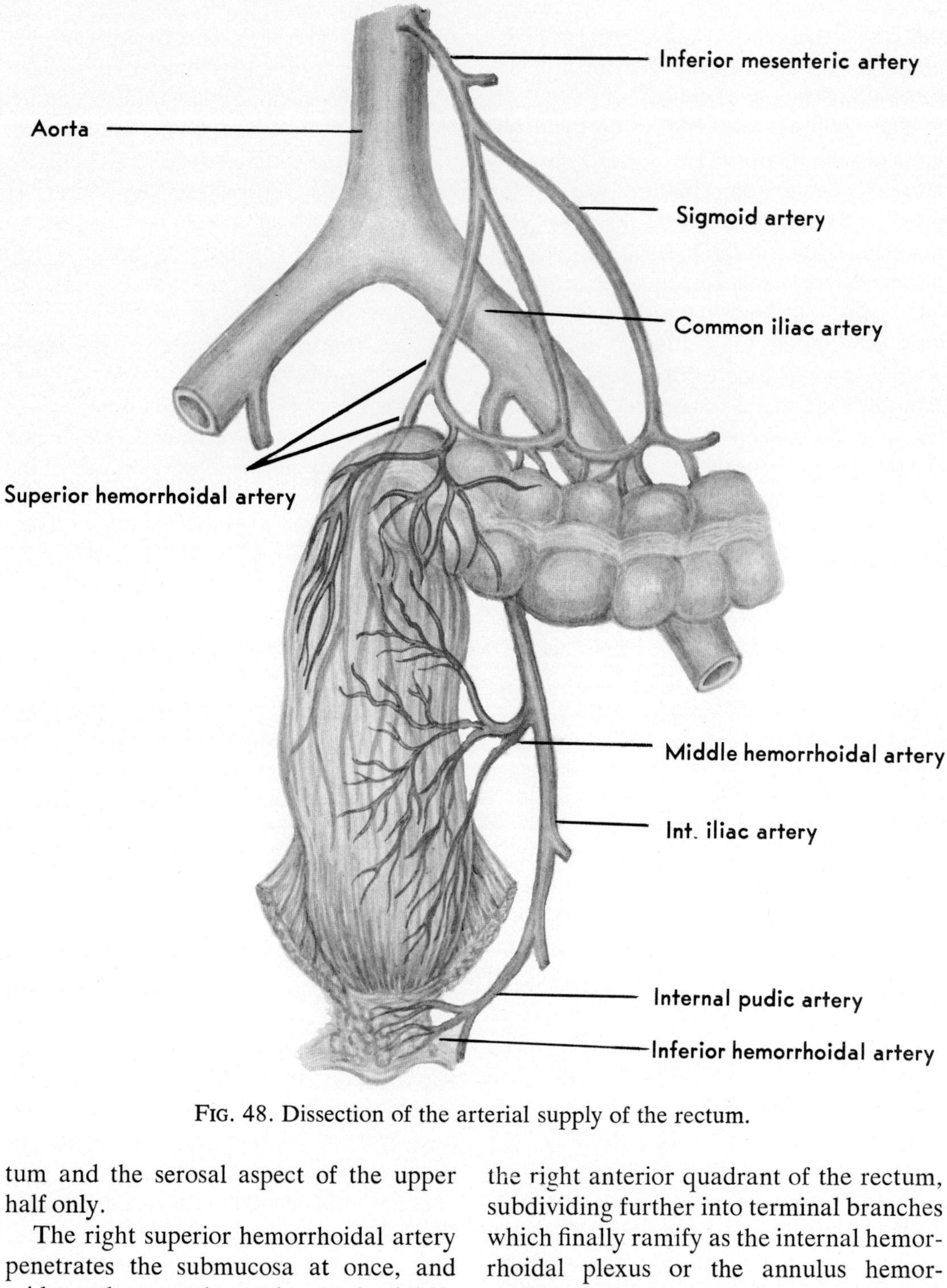

FIG. 48. Dissection of the arterial supply of the rectum.

tum and the serosal aspect of the upper half only.

The right superior hemorrhoidal artery penetrates the submucosa at once, and midway down to the anal verge it divides into two primary branches: a right anterior and a right posterior. The right anterior primary branches run downward in the right anterior quadrant of the rectum, subdividing further into terminal branches which finally ramify as the internal hemorrhoidal plexus or the annulus hemorrhoidalis of the rectum, just above the anorectal junction. It has no branches but remains a sizable vessel at the base of the columns of Morgagni at the middle of the right anterior quadrant. When its accompanying superior hemorrhoidal vein becomes varicose, this artery forms the core of the primary right anterior internal hemorrhoids, at the 11 o'clock position along the anorectal circumference with the patient in the lithotomy position.

The right posterior primary branch passes downward in the right posterior quadrant and proceeds along the right posterior quadrant. While this branch finally ends in the internal hemorrhoidal or superior hemorrhoidal plexus, it does so as a sizable vessel also at the base of the column of Morgagni at the middle or the right posterior quadrant. When the accompanying superior hemorrhoidal vein becomes varicose, this artery forms part of the primary right posterior internal hemorrhoid, located at 7 o'clock position along the anorectal circumference with the patient in the lithotomy position. During its course it gives off two secondary terminal branches, diverging from one another at right angles and ending at the right posterior commissure of the anorectal line, midway between the primary right anterior and the primary right posterior superior hemorrhoidal artery. When the accompanying veins become varicose, these secondary terminal branches become the right posterior secondary hemorrhoids (located at 6 o'clock position along the anorectal circumference with the patient in the lithotomy position), and the right lateral secondary internal hemorrhoid (located at 9 o'clock position along the anorectal circumference with the patient in the lithotomy position).

The left superior hemorrhoidal artery, after piercing the muscle coat, passes downward along the left lateral mid-plane. Like the other superior hemorrhoidal vessels, it finally ramifies as part of the internal or superior hemorrhoidal plexus, but usually as a terminal vessel it is traced in the base of the column of Morgagni at the left lateral mid-plane, forming subsequently the arterial core of the primary left lateral internal hemorrhoid when its accompanying vein becomes varicose. It also gives off two primary terminal branches which diverge from one another more or less along a straight line, passing toward each left quadrant and forming the arterial core of the secondary left anterior and the left posterior internal hemorrhoid, respectively, located at 1:30 and 4:30 o'clock positions along the anorectal circumference, midway between the commissures and the left lateral mid-plane. The primary left anterior branch also has a secondary internal hemorrhoid found in the anterior phase.

Thus, these terminals of the superior hemorrhoidal artery ramify and form the superior or internal hemorrhoidal plexus at the lower rectum at the level of the anorectal line and may even spread to the upper anal canal. These terminal arteries are located in the bases of the columns of Morgagni. Closely associated with these are the veins of the superior hemorrhoidal plexus, whose varicose dilatations are responsible for the formation of hemorrhoids. Thus we have:

Right Superior Hemorrhoidal Artery

1. Primary right anterior superior hemorrhoidal artery—first primary right anterior pile mass.

2. Primary right posterior superior hemorrhoidal artery—first primary right posterior pile mass.

2° right lateral branch . . . 2° right lateral pile mass.

2° right posterior branch . . . 2° right posterior pile mass.

Left Superior Hemorrhoidal Artery

3. Left superior hemorrhoidal artery . . . 1° left lateral pile mass.

1° left anterior superior hemorrhoidal artery . . . 2° left posterior pile mass.

2° anterior branch . . . 2° anterior pile mass.

1° left posterior superior hemorrhoidal artery . . . 2° left posterior pile mass.

What at times may appear to be tertiary hemorrhoids, at the base of the secondary hemorrhoids, are localized dilatations of nearby secondary pile masses. Thus it appears that not more than 8 hemorrhoids could be present in any given case, although enlargement of some secondary piles may appear like separate tertiary piles.

Middle Hemorrhoidal Artery

The middle hemorrhoidal arteries arise, one on each side, usually from the anterior division of the internal iliac (hypogastric artery). They may also arise from the internal pudendal as a common trunk with the vaginal and the prostatic arteries, or from the inferior vesical branch of the internal iliac artery. It runs with the corresponding vein and nerve and the areolar tissue with slips from the endopelvic fascia to form the lateral ligament or the middle neurovascular hemorrhoidal stalk of the rectum. They are generally distributed to the lower and anterior parts of the rectum in its external aspect, between the peritoneal reflection and the levator ani muscles. It also sends twigs to the base of the urinary bladder and the upper part of the vagina. Both middle hemorrhoidal arteries anastomose with each other, but the anastomoses that it forms with the superior and the inferior hemorrhoidal arteries are insignificant. This vessel generally is insignificant, although in 1 out of every 10 bodies it may be sizable enough to warrant ligation. This artery is generally conspicuous in growths affecting the middle and the lower thirds of the anterior half of the rectum. Besides varying in origin, it varies in size and distribution.

Inferior Hemorrhoidal Artery

The inferior hemorrhoidal artery primarily supplies the anal canal, but it also sends twigs to the external surface of the lower rectum. Usually it is given off as a single trunk from the internal pudendal (internal pudic) artery, as the latter lies in Alcock's canal, and pierces the medial wall of that canal and crosses the posterolateral aspect of the ischioanal space. It is accompanied by vena comites, lymphatic vessels and nerves, forming the inferior neurovascular stalk of the rectum and the anal canal. It may be supplemented by several inferior hemorrhoidal arteries which are distributed singly to the different structures usually supplied. The artery commonly divides into 4 branches:

1. **Pelvic muscular branches,** which pass posteriorly and upward to supply the obturator internus, the gluteus maximus and the levator ani muscles.

2. **Anal muscular branches,** which pass posterior to the anal canal and divide into smaller branches.

A. *Anococcygeal,* distributed to the anococcygeal ligament.

B. *Posterior sphincter,* often called the fistula artery, owing to its relation to fistulas. Usually, it is found at the 5 or 7 o'clock positions with the patient in the lithotomy position.

3. **Anterior sphincterian or anterior transverse perineal branch** usually accompanies Tuttle's anterior sphincterian nerve. It is given off just before the pudendal artery gives off the perineal artery which reaches the superficial perineal transverse

muscles. The latter is often mistaken for the anterior sphincterian or the anterior superficial perineal compartment. The anterior sphincterian artery reaches the anterior aspect of the anal canal where it gives off muscular twigs. It anastomoses freely with the anterior terminals of the lateral sphincterian branches of the inferior hemorrhoidal. It ends as small branches to the perineal body and the perianal skin.

The vascular sheaths of these vessels are presumed to direct infection to the adjacent perianal or ischioanal tissue and contribute to the causation of fistulas.

Middle Sacral Artery

The middle sacral artery arises from the back of the aorta, about 1 cm. above its bifurcation, and passes down in front of the sacrum and the coccyx, sending numerous twigs to the anococcygeal and the sacrococcygeal areas. It also sends anastomotic twigs to the inferior hemorrhoidal artery, especially the posterior sphincterian and anal muscular arteries. Usually, it ends in Luschka's coccygeal glomus (see Fig. 81 A to D).

SURGICAL CONSIDERATIONS OF THE BLOOD SUPPLY OF THE COLON AND THE RECTUM

A thorough knowledge of the vascular supply of the colon and the rectum is essential for those undertaking surgery of this part of the intestinal tract, especially in this era of radical and extended lymphadenectomies for malignant lesions. Operations on the colon and the rectum are dangerous because of the septic nature of their contents. In addition, it has that added peril of leakage at anastomoses or gangrene of a segment resulting from the compromise of its blood supply. Therefore, it is our purpose to present the more salient points in the vascular supply of the colon and the rectum from anatomic facts as applied in surgery, without detailing the operations, which is beyond the scope of this book.

The colon and its blood supply have been roughly likened to a rubber-tired wheel with a few irregularly placed spokes, which are the colic arteries, and the rim as the marginal arteries which supplies the colon through its terminal branches. It should be emphasized that these vessels should be clamped accurately and ligated only purposefully, lest disastrous incidents occur. Thus, a careful investigation of the vascular pattern and identification of the arteries to (and those adjacent to) a segment of bowel to be resected should be made before any attempts at resection are considered. This procedure may be carried out by transillumination, using a special transilluminator or by holding the bowel upward and mesially against the operating room lights. Obviously, this can be done only in the mobile and mobilized portions of the colon. Identification of the blood vessels may prove to be very difficult in the obese or when the bowel cannot be reasonably mobilized due to marked adhesions. In such cases, a knowledge of the approximate locations of vessels and feeling for their pulsations will usually suffice to establish their situations.

Mobilization of the right and the left vertical limbs of the colon is begun by incising the thickened peritoneum on each lateral gutter, which represents the line of fusion between the parietal and the visceral peritoneum. It can be cut with impunity and is referred to as the avascular line of Monk. Similarly, the right colic or hepatic flexure and the left colic or splenic flexure are mobilized by cutting their numerous peritoneal attachments, although on the left, division of the phrenicocolic ligament may result in troublesome bleeding and require ligation. The proximity of the spleen makes it vulnerable to injury, which in a few instances have required its removal. Such injuries usually are inflicted by long retractors held by the assistant who, because of the disadvantage in his position, is apt to plow into the organ when bleeding occurs. Adequate exposure through a large incision, sufficient protective covering over the spleen, and the use of retractors of appropriate size will prevent such mishaps.

The bowel may be further mobilized medially by blunt and sharp dissection to expose the more centrally located major vessels, thus permitting their early ligation prior to handling of the tumor and preventing dissemination of cancer cells through the venous drainage. Mobilization of the colon also facilitates application of heavy-gauge gauze around the tumor, which is an added means of preventing recurrence of cancer by seeding in the peritoneal cavity or in the wound.

Pertinent to the blood supply of the

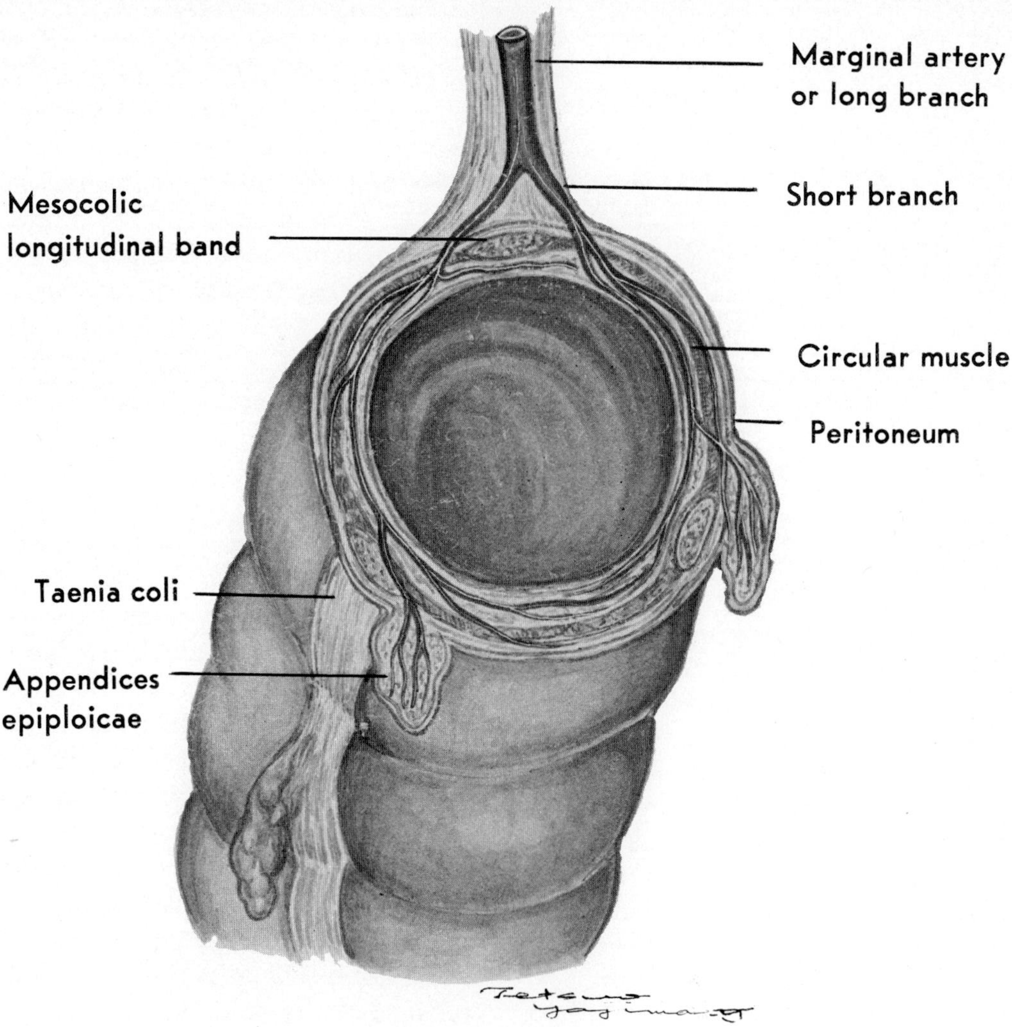

FIG. 49. Arterial blood supply of the large bowel (cross section).

colon and the rectum, inadequate mobilization of the bowel might lead to disastrous consequences. Blood vessels may be subjected to undue pull or tension and angulation because they lie beneath a loose peritoneum which allows considerable mobility and hence give a false sense of security with regard to the effect on the blood vessels. The marginal and the terminal arteries are particularly susceptible to the effects of tension that may be manifested by ischemia and/or gangrene of the areas supplied by them.

The problem of inadequate blood supply arises commonly in low anterior anastomosis and is evidenced by the high percentage of leaks in such cases. This is accounted for by the technical difficulty of placing sutures accurately and by insufficient mobilization of the proximal bowel to bring down to the rectum, tightly hugging the pelvic wall. Similarly, if the proximal end of the bowel is forcefully pulled through the anal sphincters in pull-through operations with resultant injury to the marginal arteries, sloughing of the bowel and consequent poor results are obtained.

An inadequate slack in the segment of the colon that is brought out for a colostomy and fixed to one or more layers of the abdominal wall is inviting trouble for the same reason of undue tension on the blood vessels and a compromising of blood supply.

Ligation of the main colic arteries presents no problem in the light of our experience, although it is possible to compromise the blood supply to a segment of bowel if anomalies of the vascular pattern are present. It is not to be construed that identification of blood vessels should not be undertaken. One should remember that each individual has his own vascular pattern. Hence, it is not too infrequent that the middle colic artery is ligated accidentally, and no ill effects follows. Yet there are a few instances where they are followed by gangrene of a segment of bowel. If the artery is ligated knowingly because of injury to it, the bowel should be watched for any color changes and handled accordingly.

High ligation of the inferior mesenteric artery at its origin from the aorta is a safe procedure and permits wider horizons for radicality in the dissection. This is due to the so-called marginal artery which is formed from branches of arteries that supply the colon, namely, the end of the superior mesenteric artery and adjacent branch of the ileocolic, the right colic, the upper and the lower left colic, and sigmoidal branches of the inferior mesenteric artery, and the superior hemorrhoidal artery, which is the continuation of the latter. Therefore, it extends from the distal ileum to the distal pelvic colon. The distance of the marginal artery from the margin of the colon varies from ½ cm. to several centimeters, being closest to the descending and the pelvic colon. It should be left intact when resection for a nonmalignant lesion is done, thus ensuring the colon of proximal and distal blood supply.

In the region of the splenic flexure the marginal arteries are running almost parallel with one another owing to the acute flexion of the bowel. Hence, if resection of this part is contemplated, the area must be well mobilized, and the resection is begun on its lateral aspect, never on the medial side, because the marginal arteries might be injured at points proximal to the site of resection.

When performing a colostomy, the marginal artery should always be left intact, and adequate mobilization should be made to allow exteriorization of the bowel without undue pull on the vessels. If an opening is made in the mesocolon for pur-

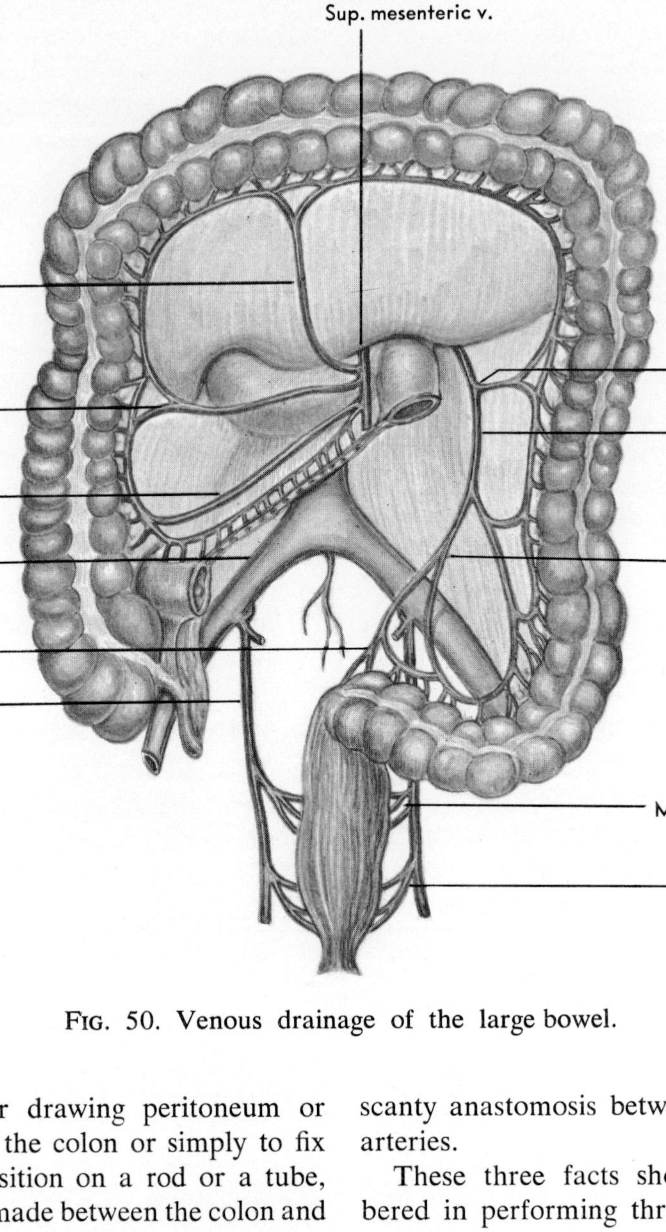

FIG. 50. Venous drainage of the large bowel.

poses of either drawing peritoneum or fascia beneath the colon or simply to fix the loop in position on a rod or a tube, the opening is made between the colon and the marginal artery. This may necessitate division of some terminal arteries.

The distribution of terminal arteries of the colon presents certain peculiar anatomic facts: (1) the subserosal position of the long arteries before they pass beneath the two amesocolic taenia to supply the relatively avascular third amesocolic portion of the colon, (2) the greater vascular supply to the mesocolic two thirds of the bowel, and (3) the comparatively scanty anastomosis between the terminal arteries.

These three facts should be remembered in performing three common procedures.

1. When clamping fat tabs, the epiploic appendage should not be pulled out so as to overstretch its attachment, and the clamp should be applied tangentially to the colonic wall. Improper handling may lead to injury to the long terminal arteries which are located in the subserosal layer before they pass beneath the longitudinal muscle to the amesocolic section of the bowel wall.

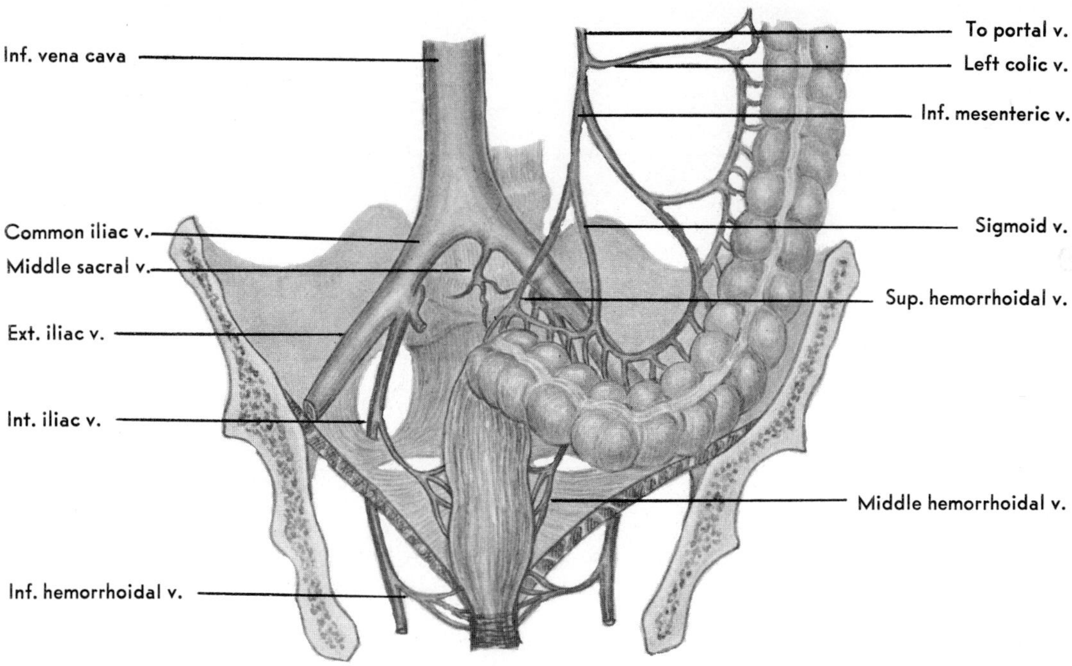

FIG. 51. Venous drainage of the sigmoid and the rectum.

2. The bowel should be cut at an acute angle (less than 45°) so that the distal and the proximal ends of the bowel have almost equal diameter. The clamp is placed in such a manner that more of the vascular mesocolic portion of the colon is retained than the amesocolic side. If the bowel is cut across perpendicular to its long axis, the long terminal branches to the amesocolic portion may be included, thus compromising the blood supply to it.

3. Incisions on the colon are made on the anterior taenia in a longitudinal fashion, the length of which should be approximately the diameter of the sigmoidoscope to be used. The incision may be closed either transversely or horizontally in 2 layers. The completeness of the muscular layer on the taenia gives ample support to the suture line.

VENOUS DRAINAGE OF THE COLON

The venous drainage of the colon starts as an intramural venous plexus which emerges as small colic veins accompanying the straight branches of the colic arteries in the mesocolic border of the bowel. These colic veins unite with others to form longer veins that follow the arterial architecture and nomenclature. The venous pattern follows closely the arterial network for the right hemicolon, providing usually an ileocolic vein, a right colic vein and a middle colic vein, which commonly unite to form a common trunk, the superior mesenteric vein. The last lies to the right and follows closely the superior mesenteric artery to its point of origin. It unites with the inferior mesenteric vein, the splenic vein, the right gastroepiploic vein, the coronary vein and the pyloric vein to form the portal vein. The manner of formation of the portal vein is subject to many variations.

The left hemicolon is drained by the sigmoidal and the left colic veins that empty into the inferior mesenteric vein. This inferior mesenteric vein passes to the left of the inferior mesenteric artery; thus,

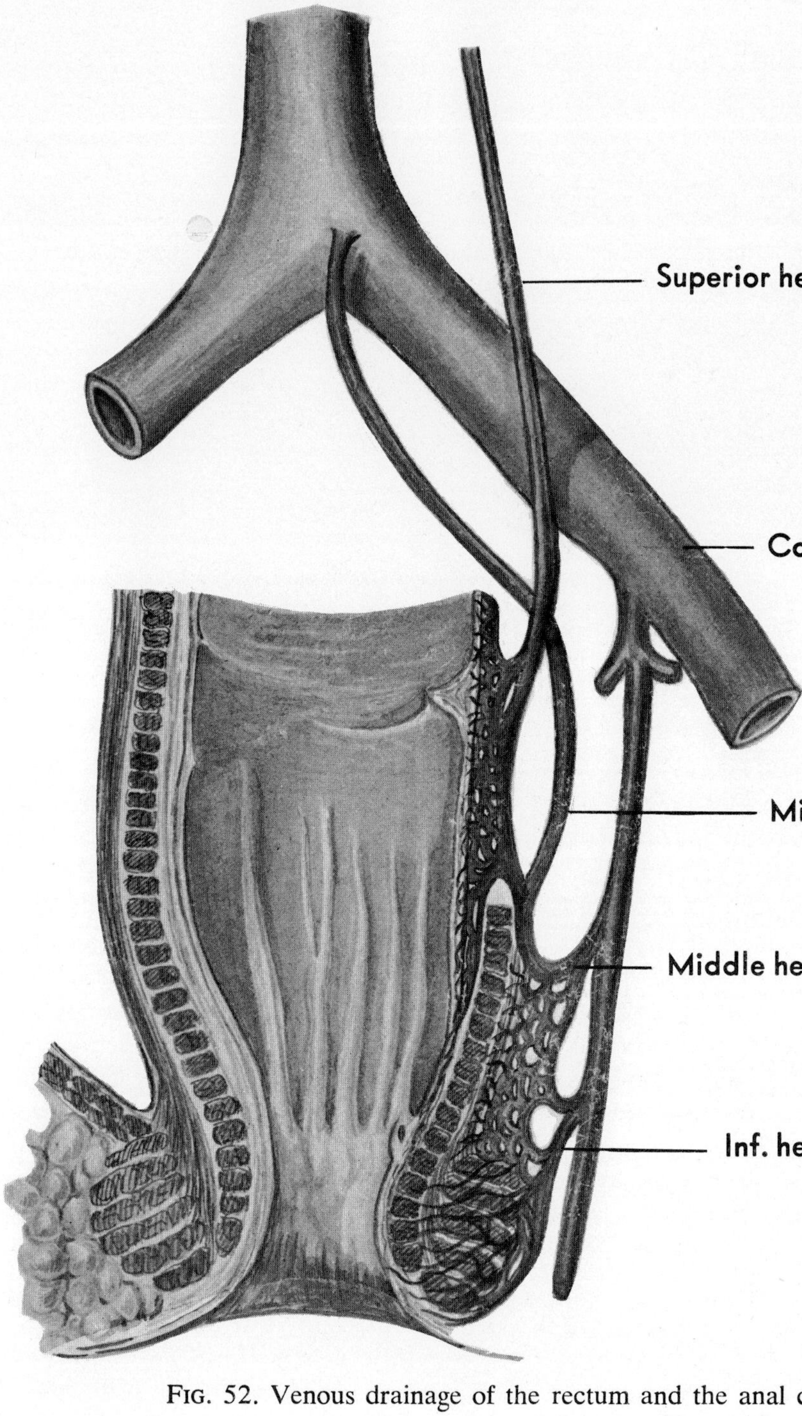

FIG. 52. Venous drainage of the rectum and the anal canal.

both mesenteric veins lie lateral to their corresponding mesenteric arteries. It then courses upward and starts to diverge from the artery until at the level of the aortic origin of the latter, where it is usually 1 to 2 cm. away. The inferior mesenteric pedicle must be ligated separately whenever aortic ligation of the inferior mesenteric artery is performed. The inferior mesenteric vein passes further upward,

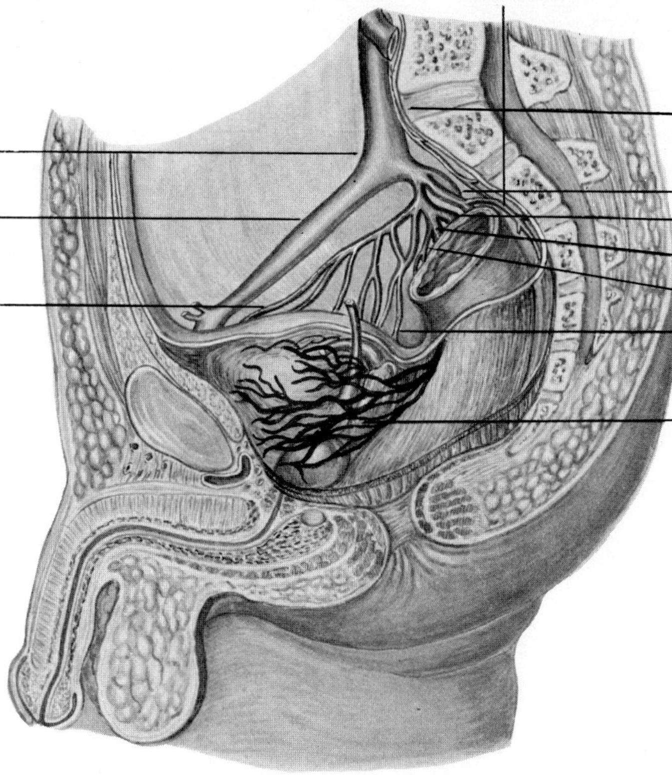

FIG. 53. Venous drainage of the pelvic viscera (male).

lying lateral to the duodenojejunal fossa hidden in the peritoneal fold that forms its upper and lateral boundary. It then curves to the right above the duodenojejunal flexure and passes behind the pancreas, where it usually joins the splenic vein to form the portal vein with the other vessels further on. In some cases it may empty directly into the superior mesenteric vein instead, either down to or at some distance from the junction of the latter with the splenic vein.

Thus both hemicolons ultimately drain into the portal vein. This is where the small bowel also drains.

VENOUS DRAINAGE OF THE RECTUM AND THE ANAL CANAL

The rectum and the anal canal are drained by a plexiform network of veins which is divided into (1) internal venous plexus, composed of submucosal vessels in the rectum and the anal canal comprising essentially the superior hemorrhoidal plexus (internal hemorrhoidal plexus); and (2) external venous plexus composed of extramural vessels of the rectum and the anal canal, essentially the same as the inferior hemorrhoidal plexus (external hemorrhoidal plexus).

The latter plexus is located in the loose perirectal tissue and, through the middle hemorrhoidal plexus, are related anteriorly to the vesicoprostatic plexus in males and the uterovaginal plexus in females. There are three distinct networks in these plexuses—superior, middle and inferior, each of which is related to the corresponding hemorrhoidal or rectal artery. The veins of the superior and the inferior groups intercommunicate with

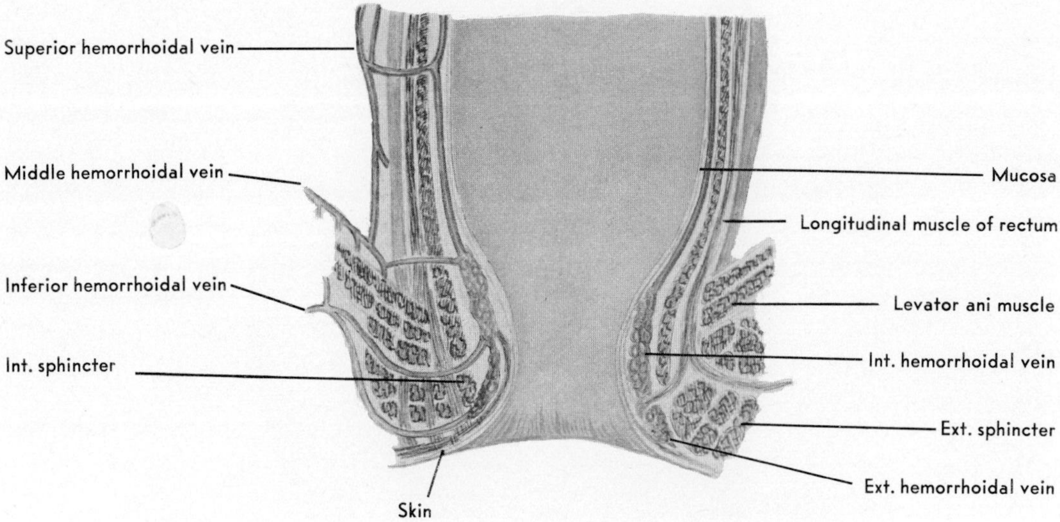

FIG. 54. Showing relations of the hemorrhoidal veins and the muscles.

one another, but those of the middle group have minimal anastomoses with each other and with the other networks.

The superior or internal hemorrhoidal plexus is located in the submucous space of the rectum and is derived from the submucosal venules between the crypts of Morgagni. They are more or less valveless, dilated vessels that end in distinctly sacculated veins. From the upper end of the superior hemorrhoidal plexus arise about 6 to 7 parallel main trunks. These pass from the bases of the columns of Morgagni, accompanied by a terminal branch of the inferior mesenteric artery and incidentally form the basis for the production of internal hemorrhoids. They pass upward and communicate freely with one another, forming the superior hemorrhoidal plexus. In their course, they receive numerous anastomotic twigs, forming a rich intercommunication with one another. Finally, two superior hemorrhoidal veins, one from each side, unite behind the rectum, accompanying the superior hemorrhoidal arteries, and form part of the superior neurovascular stalk of the rectum, which passes upward as the inferior mesenteric vein. It courses to the left of the inferior mesenteric artery, finally adding to the formation of the portal vein as previously outlined. The superior hemorrhoidal plexus drains the entire interior of the upper rectum and the upper half of the perirectal area.

The middle hemorrhoidal plexus is arranged as a network of veins outside the rectum above the level of the levator ani muscles. This begins as small submucosal vessels in the rectal ampulla, and to a small extent drains the mucosa of the middle of the rectum. It drains mainly the muscular coat and the external wall of the rectum from the level of the levator ani to the peritoneal reflection and communicates with the vesicoprostatic plexus or uterovaginal plexus. Anteriorly, this venous network ends in two or more middle hemorrhoidal veins that course laterally, forming part of the lateral stalks or the middle hemorrhoidal neurovascular stalk of the rectum, finally emptying into the internal iliac veins. Occasionally, they may empty into the inferior vesical veins or the internal pudendal veins. This middle hemorrhoidal plexus has been credited as the possible source of malignant emboli that result in local or extensive recurrences after what appears to be an extensive and adequate resection of the lower rectum.

The inferior hemorrhoidal plexus is in the perianal space of Milligan. It lies in the subcutaneous portion of the external anal sphincter and forms the marginal venous trunk which receives numerous small branches from the lower two thirds of the anal canal and the external sphincters. From this plexus, subcutaneous efferents pass anteriorly, along the cruroscrotal groove to join the internal saphenous vein at Scarpa's triangle. The more important efferents pass between the superficial and the deep parts of the external anal sphincter and proceed (1) posteriorly to join the venous plexus at the region of the coccyx, accompanying the anal muscular branches of the inferior hemorrhoidal artery; (2) laterally, as several larger veins which traverse the ischioanal space as part of the inferior neurovascular stalk, together with the inferior hemorrhoidal artery and vein. As a rule, they empty into the internal pudendal vein, which in turn is a tributary of the internal iliac vein.

From the superior hemorrhoidal plexus arise the internal or mucosal piles, while

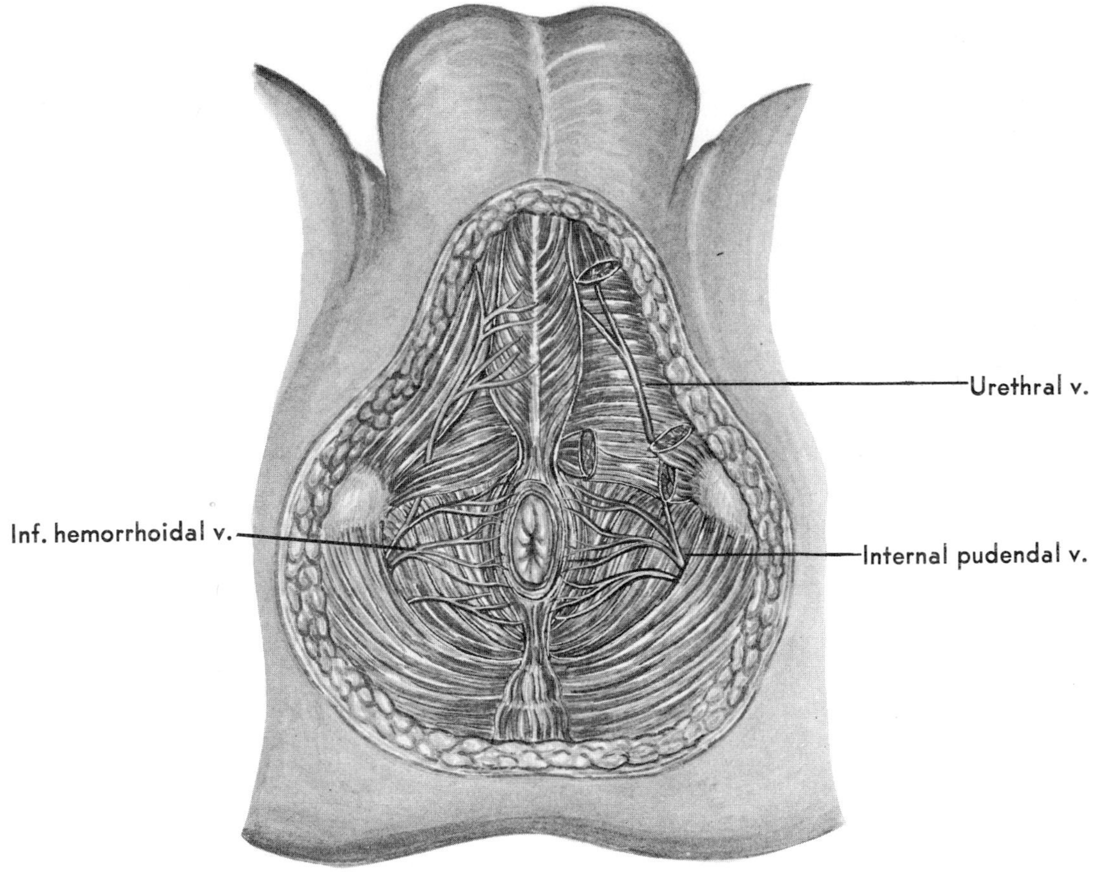

FIG. 55. Venous drainage of the male perineum.

the external or skin-covered piles arise from the inferior hemorrhoidal plexus. Thrombotic external piles generally involve the small veins running from the anal canal to the margin of the inferior hemorrhoidal plexus.

Numerous communicating veins exist between the 3 venous plexuses but principally between the external or inferior hemorrhoidal plexus (a part of the caval venous system) and the internal or superior hemorrhoidal plexus (a part of the portal venous system). This is one of the collaterals utilized during portal venous obstruction and explains the occurrence of piles in portal hypertension. By the same token, portal pyemia could occur from badly infected external piles. Congestion and thrombosis in either plexus is reflected or transmitted to the other.

SURGICAL CONSIDERATIONS OF VENOUS DRAINAGE OF COLON AND RECTUM

The venous system is one of the routes by which cancer cells disseminate. Numerous studies have been conducted that emphasize the role of venous spread, for example massaging the tumor (simulating handling of the tumor during an operation) and obtaining venous blood from the veins that drain the area. Not only has the

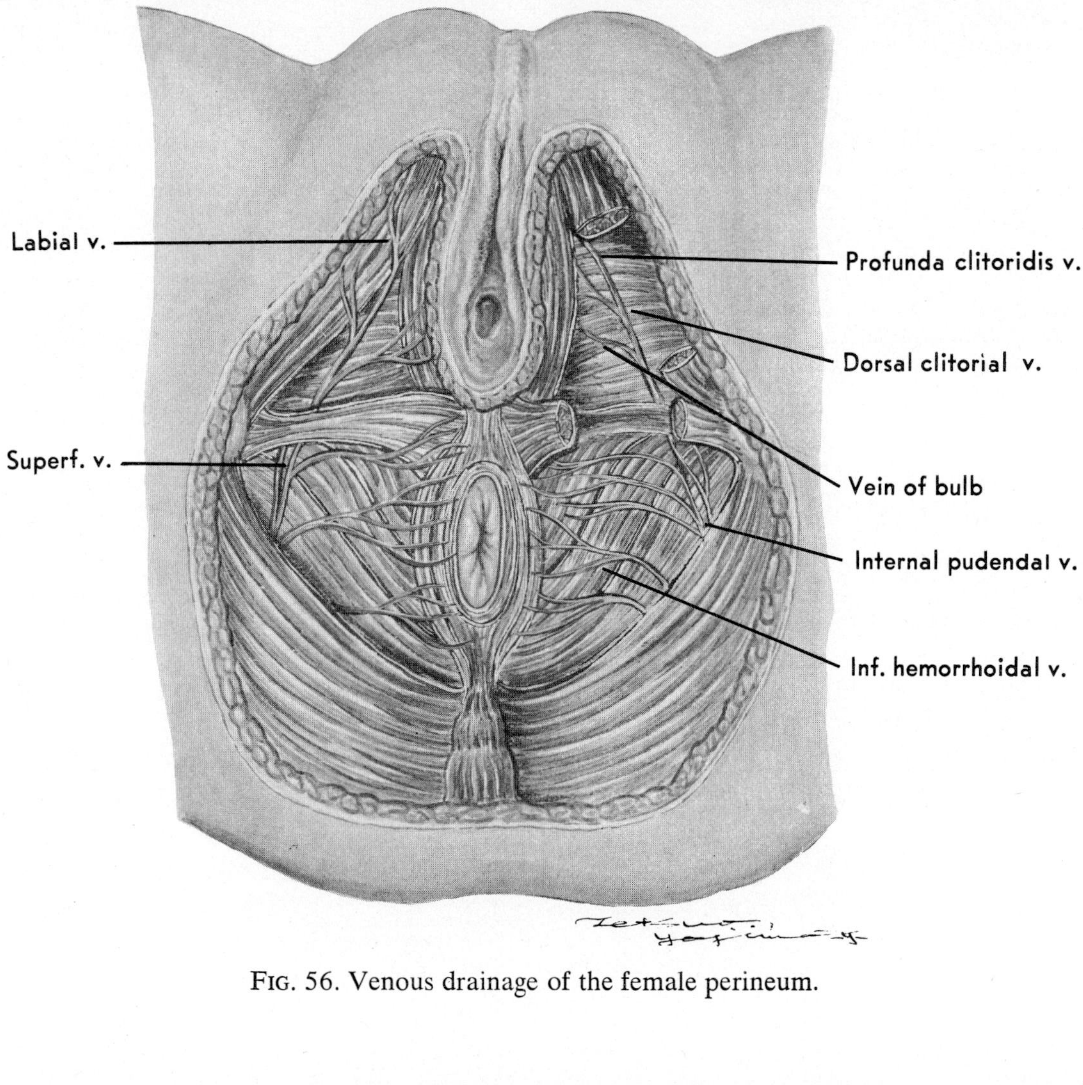

FIG. 56. Venous drainage of the female perineum.

number of circulating cancer cells been found to be increased, but more significant is the finding of clumps of tumor cells. Consequently, early ligation of the vein draining a tumor site has become a standard procedure, whenever possible, before mobilization of the involved segment of bowel is carried out. The inferior mesenteric vein is exposed by making an incision along the avascular line of Monk on the lateral side of the left colon, and by blunt and sharp dissection the bowel is freed and retracted mesially and held upward. The left ureter is identified with the gonadal vessels, and the inferior mesenteric vein will be found in the mesentery medial to the ureter. Then it is tied with heavy braided silk at a high level.

Hemorrhoidectomy, like a herniorrhaphy, is given to the novice, since it is considered a minor operation. Yet both operations have tested the skill even of experts, so that in truth no one can honestly say that he has had no failures or complications. In addition to the removal of hemorrhoidal tissue, attention should be focused on the means by which complications can be prevented. Thus, complete hemostasis must be secured by ligation of bleeders or cauterization of oozing vessels. As added security, the hemorrhoidal pedicle and the adjacent mucous membrane should be sutured to the tissue overlying the subcutaneous portion of the external sphincter muscle. The skin that is excised should be well beyond the anal verge to afford good drainage. When several hemorrhoidal masses are present, an adequate amount of mucous membrane should be left in between the wound. Oversolicitous removal of hemorrhoids and anoderm is the cause of anal stenosis which is commonly encountered. To prevent formation of skin tags, the excess or redundant anal skin should be excised, and firm pressure dressings should be applied at the conclusion of the operation.

LYMPHATIC DRAINAGE OF THE LARGE BOWEL

The general architectural pattern for lymphatic drainage of both the small and the large bowels is more or less identical. The richness of the lymphatic drainage varies among the different portions of the large bowel, decreasing in approximately the following order—ceco-appendiceal region, rectum, sigmoid, colic flexure, ascending colon, and then the descending portion of the colon.

The lymphatic drainage of the colon is composed of 3 discrete intercommunicating plexuses which drain centripetally.

1. **Intramural plexus,** composed mainly of lymphatic spaces intercommunicating with their lymphatic capillaries: (a) mucosa—lymphatic spaces are found between Lieberkühn's glands; (b) submucosa—lymphatic follicular aggregates; (c) intermuscular, between the longitudinal and the circular muscles; (d) subserosal, just beneath the serosa in those areas invested with peritoneum represented, in the extraperitoneal rectum, by a lymphatic sinus between the muscle coat and the perirectal fat. Apparently, the 3 intramural plexuses empty into the subserosal plexus through short radial channels.

The different intramural plexuses form complete networks in each layer around the bowel. They communicate with one another through the radial channels. They also communicate with the plexuses of the segments of the bowel above and below them. The communications above and below are not as abundant as those all around, as evidenced by more rapid circumferential spread compared with the longitudinal extension of the neoplasm.

The submucosal plexus in the anal canal is continuous with that of the subcutaneous lymphatic plexuses of the perianal skin. Involvement of the intramural lymphatic plexus results in Duke's Type A or Stage 1 cancer of the colon or the rectum.

2. **Intermediary plexus,** composed of valved collecting afferent lymphatic vessels that connect the intramural with the extramural lymphatics. As long as this group is not involved, the neoplasm is fairly well localized. Involvement of the intermediary plexuses only will result in Duke's Type A or Stage 2 cases in cancer of the colon or the rectum.

3. **Extramural plexus** refers essentially to the different extramural lymph nodes with their connecting channels: (a) epiploic nodes, found subperitoneally along the wall or related to the bases of the appendices epiploicae, and generally abundant along the mesocolic bands; (b) paracolic nodes, found along the short terminal branches of the marginal artery in the mesocolon, located in the medial aspects of the ascending and the descending limbs of the colon, while in the transverse colon they are found above and below it, between the two leaves of the transverse mesocolon; (c) intermediate nodes, located between the vascular arcades and the principal branches of the superior and the inferior mesenteric artery that supply the corresponding segment of the colon that is being drained; (d) proximal or central (chief or aortic) nodes, found close to the point of origin of the arteries from the aorta.

Normally, a graduated centripetal flow of lymph occurs by permeation, so that lymph passes from the intramural to the intermediary plexus and involves in succession the epiploic, the paracolic, the intermediary and finally the chief nodes. Under pathologic conditions, especially in neoplasm of the flexures, embolism may be responsible for the spread of the disease process directly from the epiploic and the paracolic nodes to the center or proximal nodes, bypassing entirely the intermediate nodes. This is referred to as "skip metastases" and must be recognized by performing a wider area of resection for neoplasms of the bowel. In other instances, direct lymphatic trunks bypassing these nodes have actually been demonstrated to pass from the epiploic and the paracolic nodes to the central nodes.

By the same token, when more proximal nodes are involved in advanced disease, a retrograde embolic spread may occur to involve the lymph nodes that normally would drain the nearby distal segment. This is very important in deciding the line of distal section of the bowel in cases of neoplasms. Such a type of retrograde metastasis is of special significance in malignancies involving the rectum where an attempt to preserve the anal sphincters is made.

Lymphatics of the Colon

The ceco-appendiceal region and the lower third of the ascending portion of the colon, together with the terminal 15 to 20 cm. of ileum, drain into the cecal and the appendiceal nodes (which belong to the epicolic nodes) and collectively are called the ileocecal nodes. They are located at the ileocolic angle and are connected by efferent trunks which pass to the intermediate group of the ileocolic nodes located halfway up the ileocolic artery. The main nodes are present at the origin of the ileocolic artery from the superior

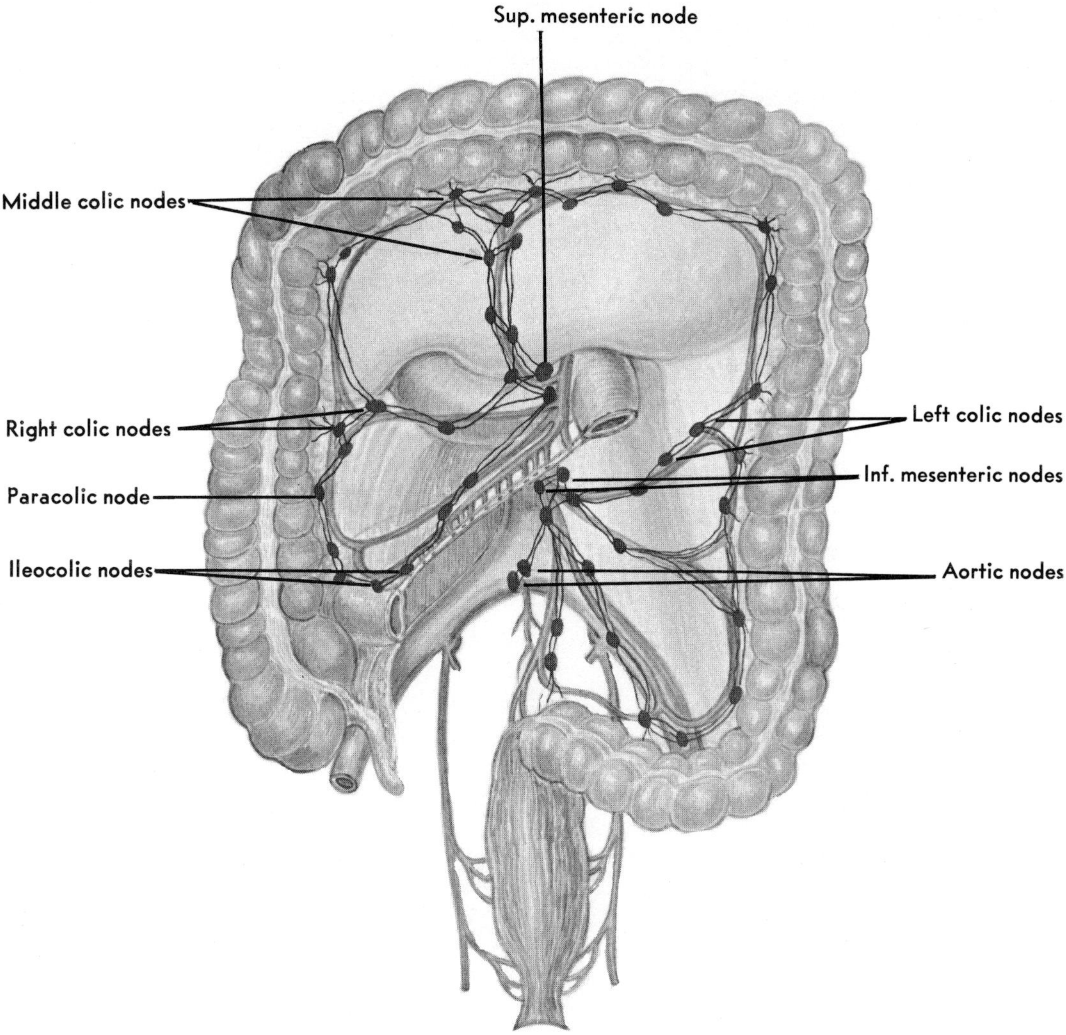

FIG. 57. Lymph drainage of the large bowel.

mesenteric artery and ultimately these empty into the root of the mesentery, forming part of the superior mesenteric system of nodes.

Lymphatic trunks have been demonstrated connecting the right ovary to the ceco-appendiceal region. These connecting trunks probably are the paths taken by cancer of the colon that becomes secondarily deposited on the right ovary.

The lymphatics of the upper two thirds of the ascending colon follow a similar pattern to the above and drain to the right colic nodes (intermediate) located along the right colic artery, which drain also at the root of the mesentery.

The lymphatics of the right colic flexure and the proximal two thirds of the transverse colon drain into the epicolic and the paracolic nodes associated with the vascular arcade of the middle colic artery. The intermediate nodes are located about the bifurcation of the middle colic artery as it enters the transverse mesocolon. They also ultimately drain into the superior mesenteric system of nodes. Efferent vessels have been demonstrated from the epicolic nodes of the right colic flexure to the gastric nodes, and from those of the transverse colon to the omental nodes.

In general, it is said that the transverse colon is better drained than the vertical segments because it has dual drainage. The flexures generally have wider drainage than any of the other segments.

The lymphatic drainage of the distal third of the transverse colon and the left colic flexure extends to the epicolic and the paracolic nodes associated with the superior branch of the left colic artery. From here two different intermediary lymphatic trunks and nodes are demonstrated:

1. Along the superior branch of the left colic to the inferior mesenteric group which lie to the left of the aorta.

2. Along the course of the inferior mesenteric vein to the superior mesenteric group of glands at the root of the mesentery.

Efferent lymphatic trunks have also been demonstrated running in the gastrosplenic ligament to the hilar nodes of the spleen.

The descending colon drains into the epicolic and the paracolic nodes associated with the descending and the ascending colic branches of the inferior branch of the left colic from the inferior mesenteric artery. The chief nodes are located with the inferior mesenteric group of nodes.

The pelvic portion of the colon drains into the epicolic and the paracolic nodes related to the terminals of the sigmoid arteries. Efferents pass to the intermediate nodes of the main sigmoid artery as it springs from the inferior mesenteric artery. The chief nodes are at the aortic origin of the inferior mesenteric artery.

Intermediate lymph nodes are also found along the accessory colic vessels. In instances when an artery has an aberrant abnormal location, the corresponding intermediary nodes and chief nodes may also be located erratically.

LYMPHATIC DRAINAGE OF THE RECTUM

The intramural lymphatic network of the rectum is very similar to that of the colon. It has mucosal, submucosal and intermuscular plexuses.

The submucosal network is continuous with that of the pelvic colon above and the lymphatics of the subcutaneous network of the anal canal below.

The intermuscular plexus is continuous with that of the pelvic colon above and the lymphatics of the external sphincter below.

The subserosal plexus in the case of the extraperitoneal rectum is found in the perirectal fat outside the longitudinal muscle.

The intramural plexus of the rectum is divided into two zones, an upper and a lower, by the middle rectal valve or the transverse rectal fold of Kolrausch. This delineation between the upper and the lower zones is distinct, which we have conclusively demonstrated experimentally. Intramural injection of dyes of different colors demonstrated the different paths of spread as outlined by the colored solution. This plica also delimits the different zones of extramural spread as outlined by the dye.

The intermediary plexus of the rectum forms an extensive intercommunication of lymphatic efferents that drain the various intramural plexuses. From the former arises the different parts of the extramural lymphatic system: the superior, the middle (lateral) and the inferior pathways. The

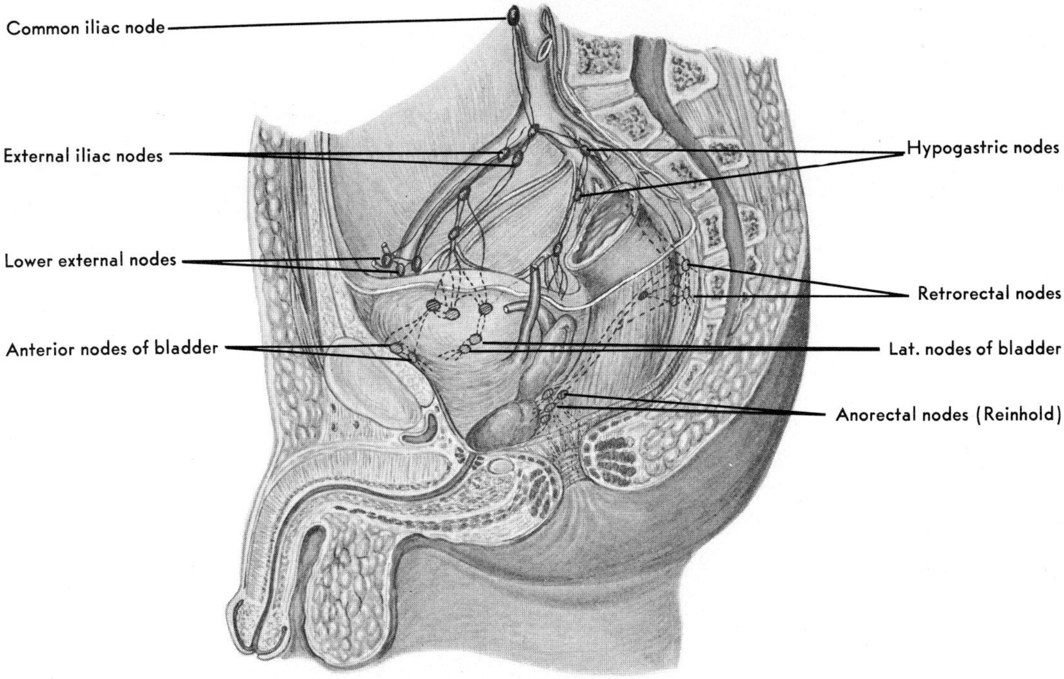

FIG. 58. Lymph drainage of the pelvic viscera (male).

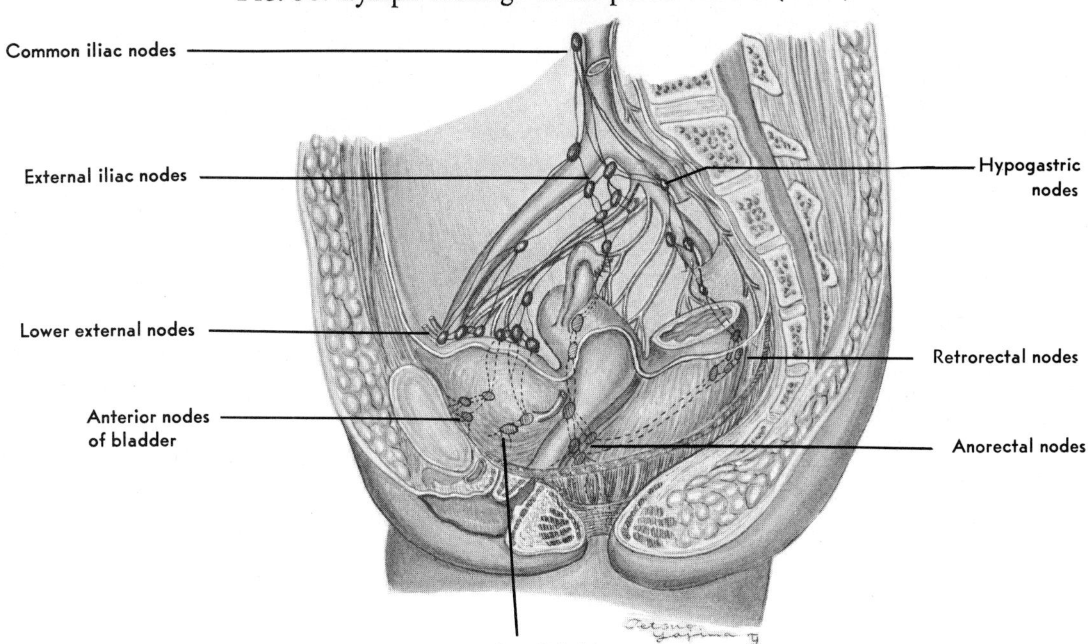

FIG. 59. Lymph drainage of the pelvic viscera (female).

so-called Gerota's nodes, which are found between the perirectal fascia and the rectum, represent part of the intramural plexus of the rectum. It drains upward and backward and also represents the superior zone of the rectum.

The superior zone is the most important and drains roughly the upper rectum and the distal colon. It drains 3 groups of discrete nodes found within the mesocolon and the mesorectum.

1. *Retrorectal nodes,* generally referred to as the sacral nodes, are found at the bifurcation of the superior hemorrhoidal arteries. They drain the main part of the upper rectum.

2. *Rectosigmoid group,* found at the junction of the sigmoidal and the superior hemorrhoidal artery; it drains the upper rectum and part of the distal colon.

3. *Rectosigmoidocolic group,* found close to the origin of the first sigmoidal artery from the left colic. These nodes can receive directly from the rectum and the sigmoid and iliac colons and therefore constitute the most important group of nodes in rectosigmoidal malignancies.

All the nodes from the superior zone finally drain into the root of the inferior mesenteric artery.

The middle or lateral zone lies in the subperitoneal tissue and ramifies throughout the complex visceral component of the endo-abdominal fascia and ultimately empty into about 6 nodes that drain into the iliac nodes. There are 3 main divisions or pedicles.

1. *The anterior pedicle of Reinhold,* which drains the lower third of the rectum, extending between the layers of the rectogenital septum and along the lateral margins of the prostate gland, the seminal vesicles, or the vaginal wall. Usually, it drains into the internal iliac nodes. Occasionally, it may drain into the external iliac group, anastomosing with the middle hemorrhoidal and the lateral sacral lymphatics.

2. *Lateral pedicle*—the most important pedicle in this group. Experimentally and by injection of dye prior to resection, we have demonstrated constantly the lymphatics following closely the middle hemorrhoidal vessels. Only in a few instances were thin lymphatics visualized between the levators and the pelvic fascia, but never was a node found in the latter location. This emphasizes the pathologic studies made by Wood and Wilkie and by Dukes who showed that the levators are not a place where metastases occur but rather are subject to direct spread. The lymphatics of the lateral pedicle drain into the obturator or internal iliac nodes.

3. *Posterior pedicle,* consisting mainly of vessels that accompany the lateral and the middle sacral vessels in the region of the promontory of the sacrum: (a) the middle sacral group, draining into the nodes located at the promontory of the sacrum; (b) the lateral sacral group, draining into those located between the bifurcation of the internal iliac and the common iliac vessels. The inferior pedicle drains the lower third of the rectum, the perianal skin and the external sphincter muscle. The efferents traverse the ischioanal fat, with the inferior neurovascular stalk, passing through Alcock's canal, finally emptying into the internal iliac nodes.

LYMPHATICS OF THE ANAL CANAL AND THE PERINEAL SKIN

Intramural Lymphatics

The intramural lymphatics of the anal canal follow the same pattern as those of the rest of the colon and the rectum.

1. **Mucosal** (actually cutaneous), lying within the lining of the modified skin or anoderm.

2. **Submucosal** (actually subcutaneous), lying beneath the anoderm, especially at the column of Morgagni.

3. **Intermuscular,** lying between the external and the internal sphincters and also related to the conjoined longitudinal muscle bundle of the rectum.

These different plexuses anastomose freely with the corresponding network of the terminal rectum above and those of the perianal region below.

Extramural Lymphatics

The extramural lymphatic system is divided into two groups:

1. **Superior group,** at the level of the anorectal line, draining the subjacent pecten, and sending out efferents that accompany the middle hemorrhoidal and the internal pudendal vessels, forming part of the middle and the inferior neurovascular stalks of the rectum.

2. **Inferior group,** lying more or less posterior to the pecten and draining into 8 to 10 afferents with those of the perianal region to the superficial inguinal nodes. The latter drain also the thigh and the anogenital fold and empty into the external iliac nodes.

There is a very rich anastomosis between the lymphatics of the terminal rectum, the anal canal and the perianal skin. This makes it difficult to trace the anatomic pathway by which a particular network of a definite area drains. The peri-

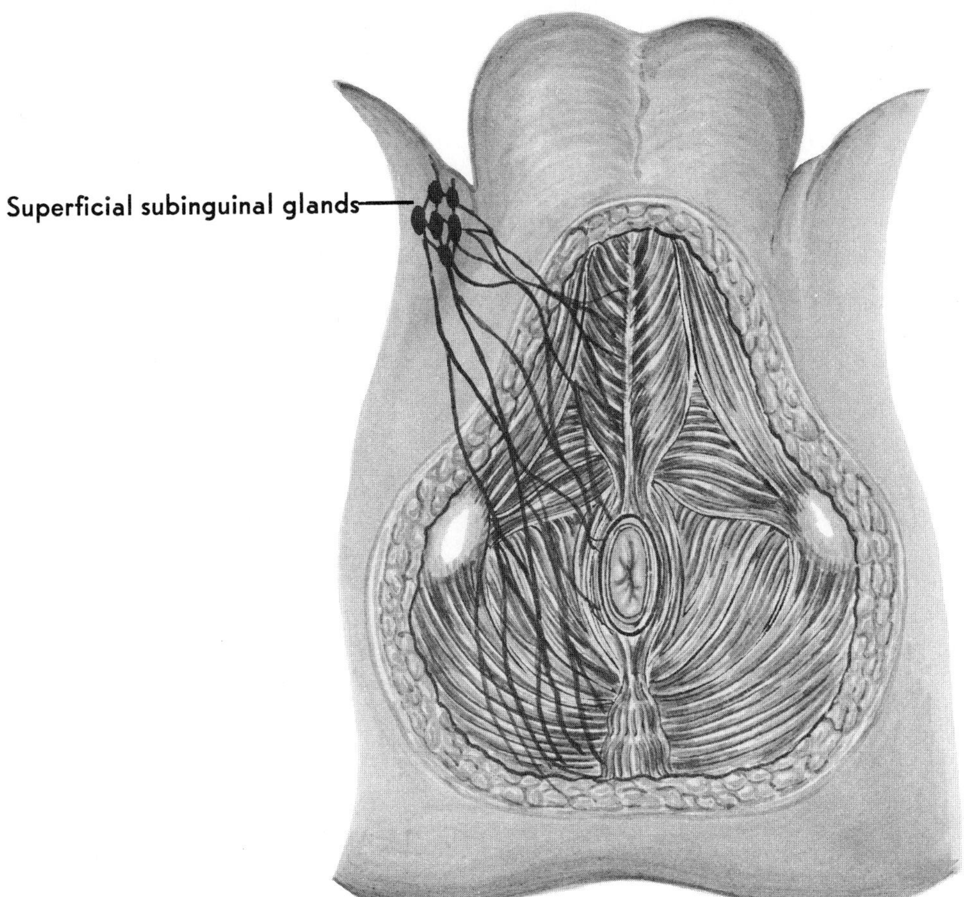

Fig. 60. Lymph drainage of the male perineum.

anal cutaneous lymphatics are divided into a superficial and a deep group. They drain the perianal skin and the superficial subjacent structures and then are carried along channels located in the perineoscrotal or labial folds, terminating in the inguinal nodes. While they generally drain into the inferolateral group of inguinal nodes, they may also drain into the inferomedial and the superomedial group of inguinal nodes.

There is an extensive anastomosis with the sacrococcygeal, the gluteal and the perianal lymphatics. Reverse lymph flow is not unusual in cases of very rich anastomosis. Nesselrod believes that Goodsall's rule of location of the internal opening of a fistula could be explained by the disposition of the perianal lymphatics. The latter are directed anteriorly along the genitocrural fold to the superficial inguinal group. The fistulae draining anteriorly have a longer tract than those opening posteriorly in relation to the center of the anal opening.

The internal iliac nodes send efferents to the common iliac group which drain into the lumbar chain of nodes, finally passing into the thoracic duct.

The superior and the inferior mesenteric lymph nodes, together with the celiac nodes, form the preaortic group of nodes. These different groups have intercommunications with one another. From this group, a major lymphatic channel, the intestinal trunk, arises and passes to the para-aortic nodes found at the left of the aorta. It ends in the lumbar trunk (14 out of 20 bodies), right lumbar trunk (1 out of 20 bodies), or directly as a third lymph duct to the thoracic duct (5 out of 20 bodies). The superior mesenteric nodes usually drain into the intestinal trunk, while in a number of cases, the inferior mesenteric nodes may drain directly into the lumbar nodes.

SURGICAL CONSIDERATIONS IN CANCER OF COLON, RECTUM AND ANAL CANAL

Based on the foregoing discussion of the lymphatics of the colon, the rectum and the anal canal, certain fundamental principles should be followed when performing an operation for "cure" of a patient with cancer. With adequate preparation of the patient, excellent anesthesia, and knowledge of fluid and electrolyte balance, a segment of colon of almost any amount can be resected safely with low morbidity and mortality. Based on present knowledge, a well-performed cancer operation would assure the patient of a good chance of long-term survival. The operation should consist of removal of the tumor, a wide margin of normal bowel, and removal of all possible areas of lymphatic drainage. The attitude of the operator should be that a malignant lesion, regardless of its size, has already metastasized to regional lymph nodes. Therefore, there should be no compromise in the extent of dissection. Our operative specimens cleared by the Spalteholz-Gilchrist technic showed 63 per cent involvement of the lymph nodes, with exclusion of cases with obvious liver metastases.

In addition to the extensive lymphatic dissection, other ancillary procedures to lower the incidence of local recurrence or widespread dissemination of cancer cells should be observed. These are early ligation of the venous return, use of tumoricidal solutions, wrapping of the tumor segment, and proximal and distal ligation of the normal bowel whenever possible. These procedures, while highly desirable, may be totally omitted if in the judgment of the surgeon they will unduly prolong the operation in the poor risk or obese patient, remembering that many patients have survived for many years without the benefit of an ideal operation.

Under optimal conditions the following resections should be observed to meet the standard of an ideal operation.

Cancer of the Cecum and the Ascending Colon

The bowel to be resected should include the distal 8 to 10 inches of ileum to the junction of the proximal and the middle thirds of the transverse colon. The ileocolic and the right colic arteries are divided at their origin from the superior mesenteric artery. The right major branch of the middle colic artery is likewise divided. This wide expanse of resection includes the lymphatics, although in the female the right ovary is also included in the resection, since lymphatic trunks have been demonstrated connecting the ovary and the ceco-appendiceal region. Since 1950 we have routinely performed a bilateral oophorectomy in all female patients under 70. Continuity of the bowel may be re-established by end-to-end anastomosis, end-to-side anastomosis, or side-to-side anastomosis. The mesentery is closed, but reperitonealization of the right lateral gutter is not essential.

Cancer of the Hepatic Flexure

This area is drained by the lymphatics along the vascular arcade of the middle colic artery, and direct efferent lymphatic channels may exist from the epicolic nodes adjacent to the bowel to the gastric and the omental nodes. Therefore, in addition to the area of resection described above, the distal transection of the bowel is made at the junction of the middle and the distal thirds of the transverse colon with inclusion of the greater omentum and the gastrocolic ligament. The middle colic artery is ligated close to its origin from the superior mesenteric artery. Re-establishment of the continuity of the bowel is carried out by any one of the methods mentioned above.

Cancer of the Midtransverse Colon

The lymph drainage of this portion of the colon is through the paracolic nodes, a large part of which goes back to the right, to the middle colic nodes and to the left, to the left colic nodes and the inferior mesenteric group. The lymph nodes in the gastrocolic ligament may also be involved. Therefore, the resection should encompass both colic flexures with the greater omentum and the gastrocolic ligament. The middle colic artery is ligated at its origin, and the left colic artery is also divided. Thus, the right colic artery and the ascending branch of the inferior mesenteric artery are preserved.

Cancer of the Splenic Flexure

Besides the usual lymph drainage pattern that occurs in this area to the nodes along the left colic artery and the main nodes around the inferior mesenteric artery and the midcolic chain on the right, lymphatic channels to the hilum of the spleen and to the nodes in the gastrocolic ligament may also be present. Owing to the inaccessibility of the region of the splenic flexure it is reasonable enough to include in the resection that segment of the bowel and its mesentery from the midtransverse colon to the mid or lower sigmoid, with ligation of the left colic artery at its origin and the left branch of the middle colic artery. An end-to-end anastomosis is performed to re-establish continuity between the transverse and the sigmoid colons.

Cancer of Descending Colon, Sigmoid, Rectum and Anal Canal

During the past decade, it has been the practice of the authors to perform high ligation of the inferior mesenteric artery with aortoileopelvic lymphadenectomy for "cure" of patients with cancer of the descending colon, the sigmoid, the rectum and the anal canal. The only exceptions to performance of the procedure are: (1) elderly patients, 65 years or more, (2) poor-risk patients who in our judgment could not tolerate prolonged surgical procedures, (3) extremely obese, (4) presence of liver metastases and (5) when obviously a curative operation is impossible. The procedure has been rewarded by improved survival rates of 5 and 10 years.

Briefly, the procedure is as follows: After the abdomen is opened through a long left paramedian incision, the requirements for a curative resection are determined. If the tumor site is in an accessible situation, the area is covered with heavy-gauge gauze, encircling the entire circumference of the bowel, and each end is tied with umbilical tape. The descending colon and the sigmoid colon are then mobilized, and the inferior mesenteric vein is ligated. The medial peritoneal incision is made from just below the third portion of the duodenum and across its inferior border to the left over the aorta. The right incision is carried downward to the medial side of the right ureter as it crosses the bifurcation of the right common iliac artery and continued down into the pelvis across the posterior aspect of the bladder (rectovesical pouch) to meet its counterpart from the left. Lymph node dissection is begun from a point below the pancreas. It is carried down over the vena cava, then on the aorta, clearing the retrocaval and the para-aortic lymphatics, including the important lateral nodes on the left side, thus exposing the psoas muscle. The inferior mesenteric artery is cleared for 1 cm. from its origin and ligated with heavy braided silk and divided. The dissection is then carried caudally, clearing the tissues around the common iliac arteries, especially those located at the bifurcation, those around the internal iliac arteries and on the promontory of the sacrum. If a Miles abdominoperineal excision is contemplated, both internal iliac arteries are ligated before mobilization of the rectum. Finally, the lymphadenectomy is carried down into the pelvis and includes the obturator nodes and the lateral ligaments.

The level of proximal transection of the bowel is determined, and particular attention is paid to the adequacy of its blood supply. Should an end-to-end anastomosis be made to re-establish continuity of the bowel, the following essentials should be established to ensure a safe anastomosis: (a) demonstrable brisk bleeding from the cut ends of the bowel; (b) adequate slack so that undue tension on blood vessels and suture line is avoided; (c) optimum exposure so that sutures may be placed accurately; and (d) if in doubt as to the integrity of the anastomosis, a transverse colostomy or cecostomy should be made as an added precaution.

NERVE SUPPLY OF THE LARGE BOWEL

The nerve supply of the colon, the rectum and part of the anal canal is derived from the autonomic nervous system. The autonomic nervous system is divided into a thoracolumbar or sympathetic pathway

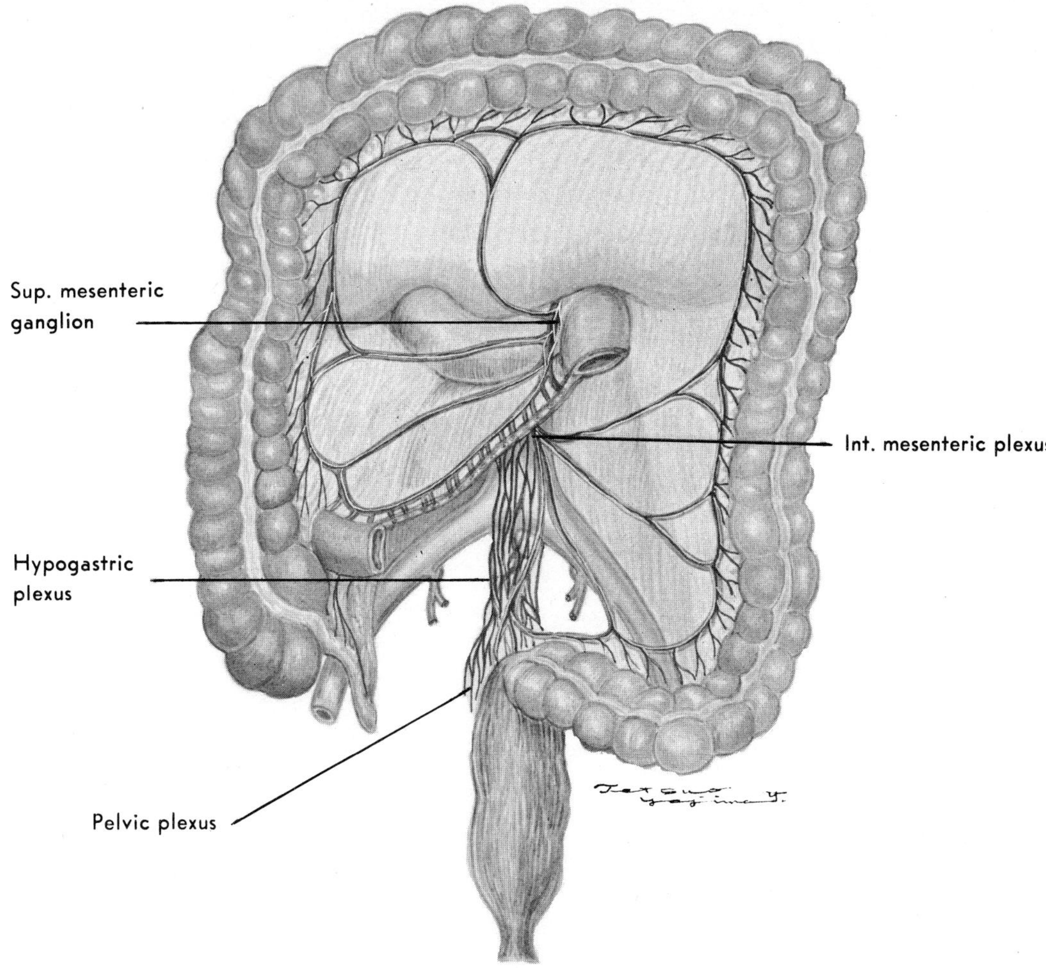

FIG. 61. Nerve supply of the large bowel.

and a craniosacral parasympathetic pathway. The basic structure of the two pathways is essentially the same—a pair of neurons which synapse in the ganglion cell. The presynaptic portion is the preganglionic fiber, while the postsynaptic portion is the postganglionic fiber. The former has a central connection, while the latter has a peripheral distribution.

SYMPATHETIC PATHWAY

The cell bodies of the preganglionic fibers of the sympathetic system are located in the intermediolateral cell columns of the gray matter of the spinal cord between the T-1 to the L-3 segments. These sympathetic preganglionic fibers leave the cord by way of the anterior (ventral) root of the spinal nerve and pass by way of the white communicating ramus to the paravertebral ganglia of the sympathetic chain. Only those fibers from T-10 to L-3 furnish the sympathetic supply to the large bowel. Fibers from T-10 to T-12 do not synapse in the sympathetic ganglia but unite to form the lesser splanchnic nerve which goes to the superior mesenteric ganglia where they synapse. On the other hand, fibers from L-1 to L-3 synapse right in the sympathetic paravertebral ganglia, and the sympathetic postganglionic fibers from the inferior mesenteric ganglion. Sympathetic postganglionic fibers from the superior mesenteric ganglia are distributed to the ascending and the transverse portions of the colon, while those of the inferior mesenteric ganglia supply the descending and the pelvic portions of the colon. Both the superior and the inferior mesenteric ganglia intercommunicate through the intermesenteric plexus at the lateral sides of the aorta. They also form a rich anastomotic network with the celiac and the aorticorenal ganglia, forming a preaortic plexus, an autonomic nerve plexus in front of the aorta.

The sympathetic postganglionic fibers

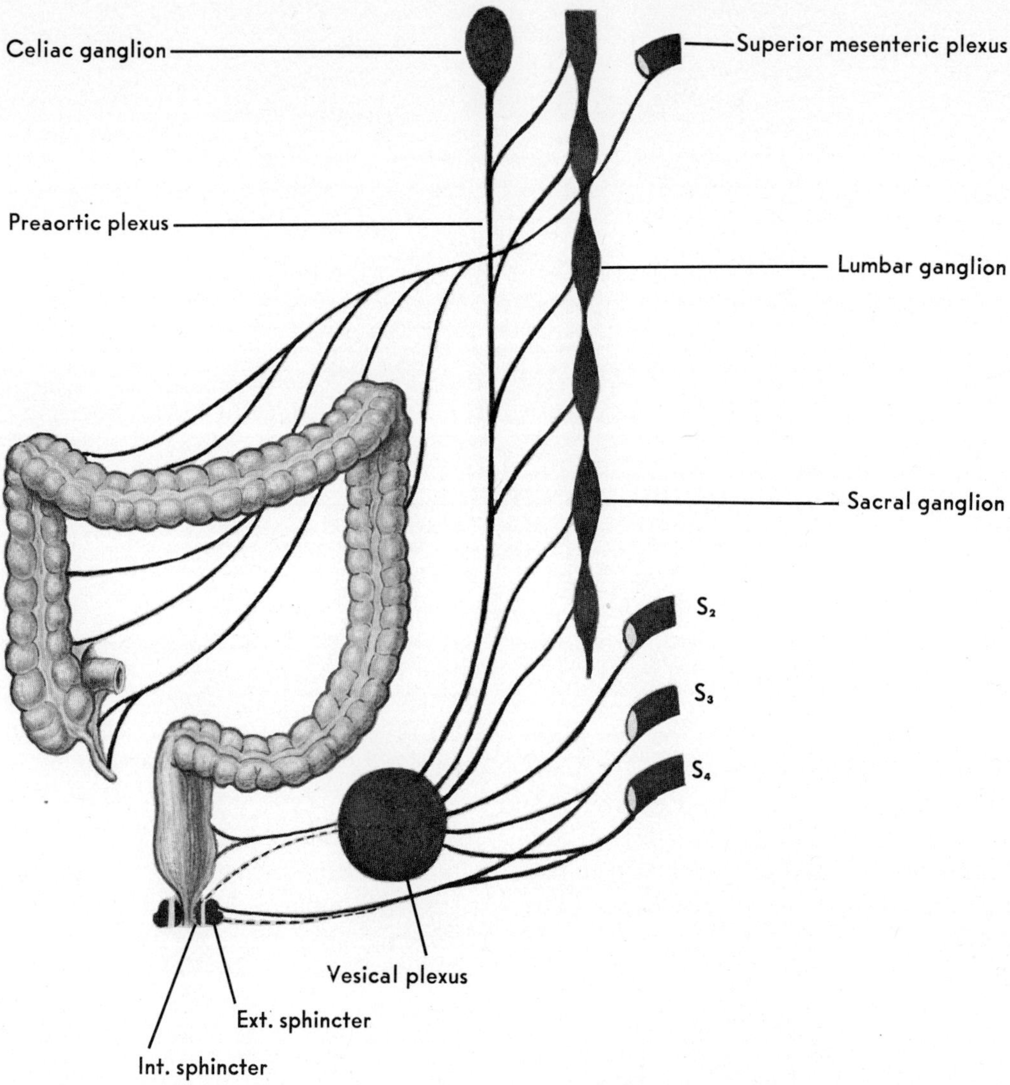

FIG. 62. Scheme of the general arrangement of the autonomic nervous system.

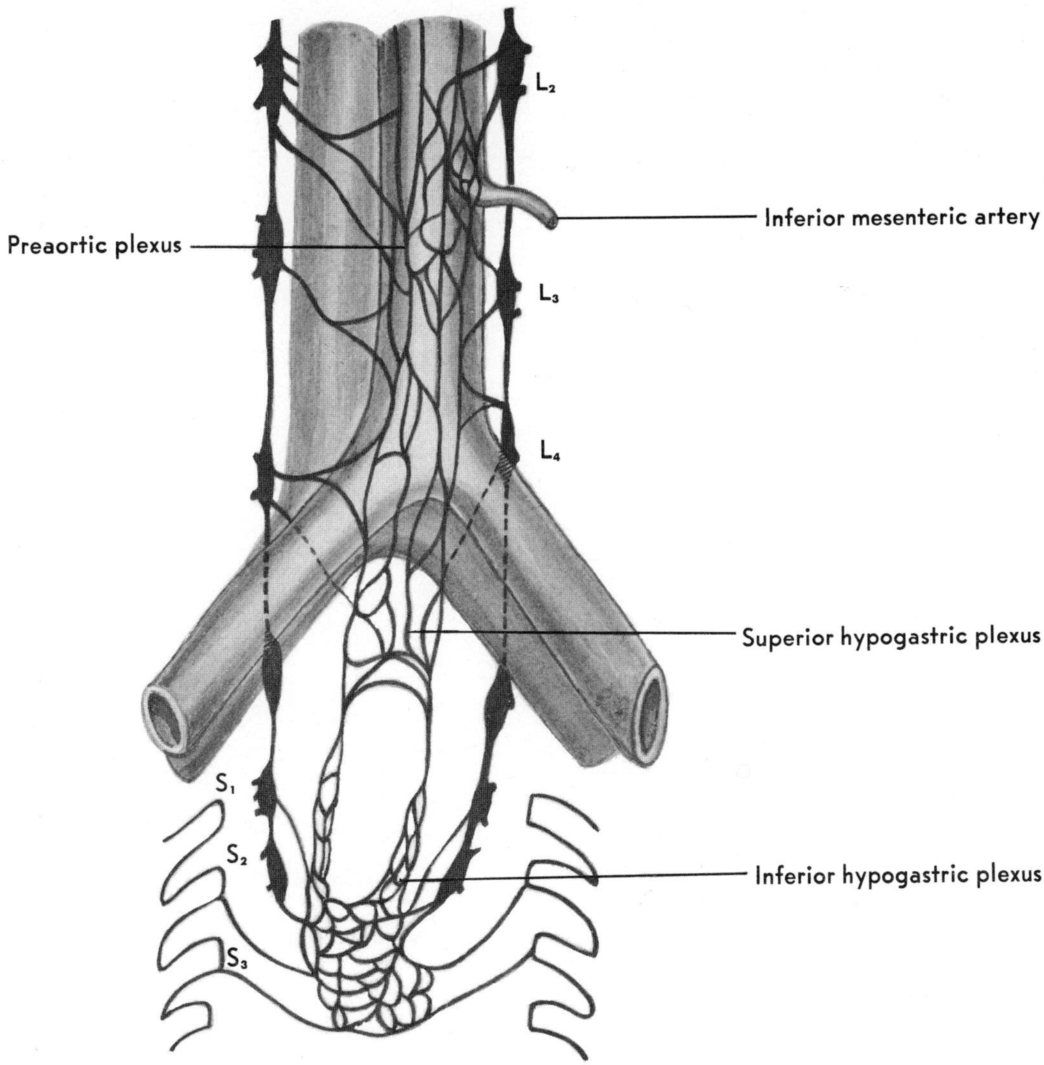

FIG. 63. Schematic drawing showing the presacral nerve.

may be distributed in any of several ways: (1) usually (10 out of 12 bodies) as a network called the hypogastric plexus; (2) as a pair of distinct hypogastric nerves (1 in 12 bodies); and (3) as a solitary presacral nerve of Latarjet (1 in 12 bodies).

The hypogastric plexus lies subperitoneally, partially embedded in the visceral endopelvic fascia of the interiliac triangle, and has been described as being composed of a superior and an inferior condensation with an inconstant middle hypogastric plexus in between. The two main condensations are connected by a pair of hypogastric nerves. The superior mesenteric plexus lies on the sacral promontory just caudad to the aortic bifurcation. From here a pair of hypogastric nerves, one on each side of the rectum, course downward and laterally behind the base of the urinary bladder where the inferior hypogastric plexus is located. The inferior hypogastric plexus sends postgan-

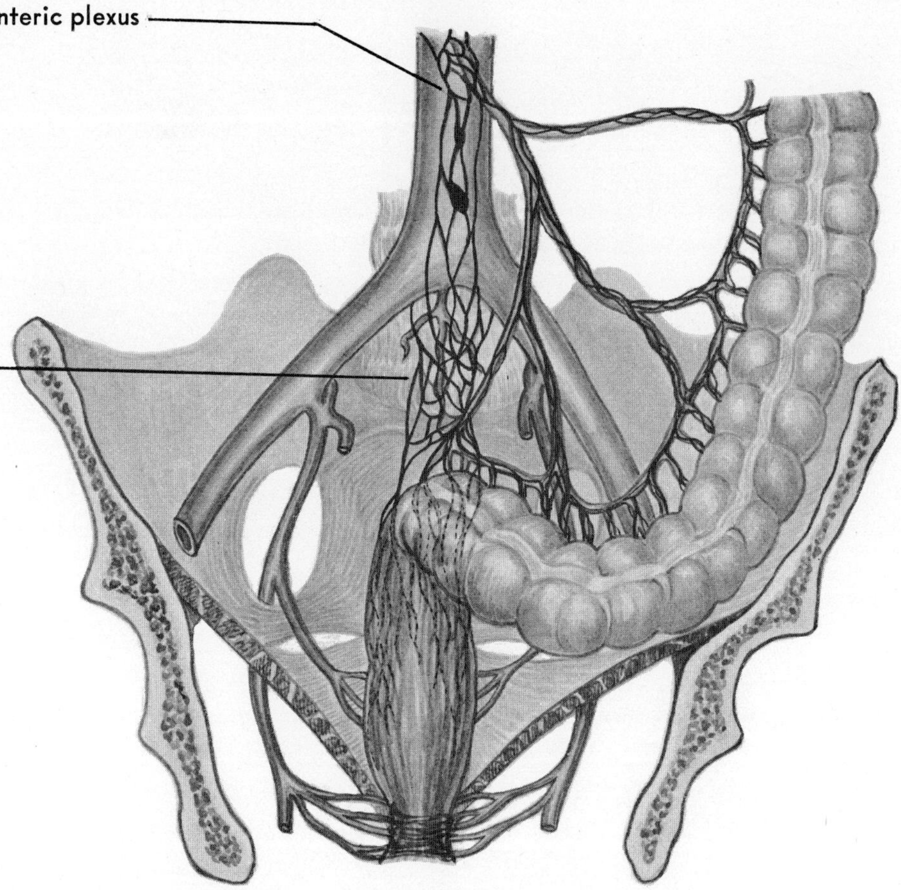

FIG. 64. Nerve supply of the sigmoid and the rectum.

glionic fibers to the rectum, the urinary bladder and the external genitalia.

The preaortic plexus also sends fibers along the wall of the branches of the aorta, the sympathetic periarterial plexus, from which fibers are distributed with the blood supply. Thus the sympathetic fibers reach the vessels, the glands and the smooth muscles of the colon through the colic arteries, and the rectum through the superior and the middle hemorrhoidal arteries. These may be identified in the subserous coat and also within the smooth muscle layer of the bowel. The sympathetic supply of the anal canal and the anorectal sphincter is distributed with the inferior neurovascular stalk.

Parasympathetic Pathway

The parasympathetic or craniosacral outflow has a dual central origin from (1) the vagus nerve and (2) the sacral portion of the spinal cord.

Preganglionic fibers from the vagal portion arise from the dorsal motor nucleus in the medulla oblongata and pass by way of the right vagus nerve to the abdomen. These fibers are distributed with the superior mesenteric plexus (of the sympathetic system) with the branches of the superior mesenteric artery to the cecum, the appendix, the ascending colon and possibly to the middle of the transverse colon. Curiously enough, this represents the postarterial segment of the midgut.

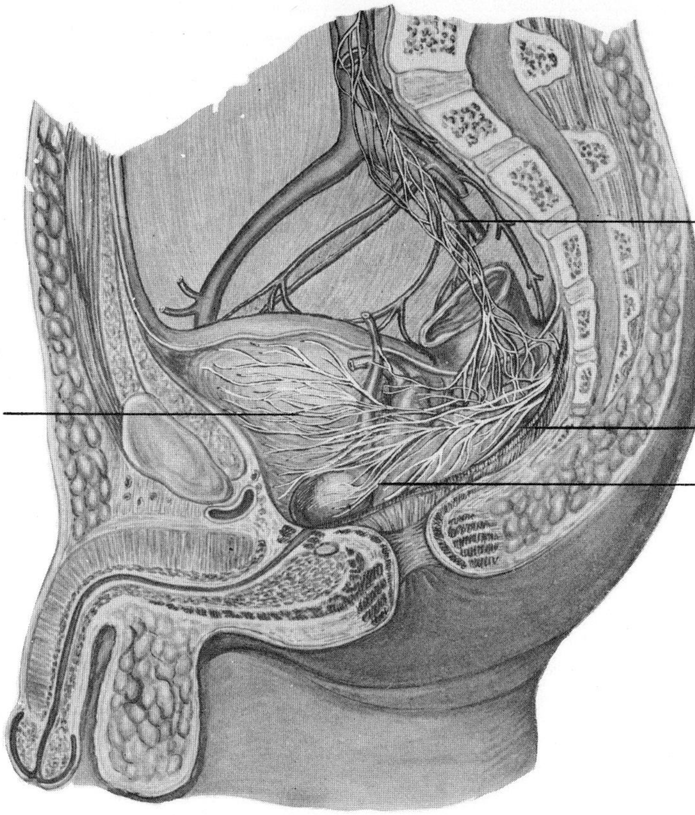

FIG. 65. Nerve supply of the pelvic viscera (male).

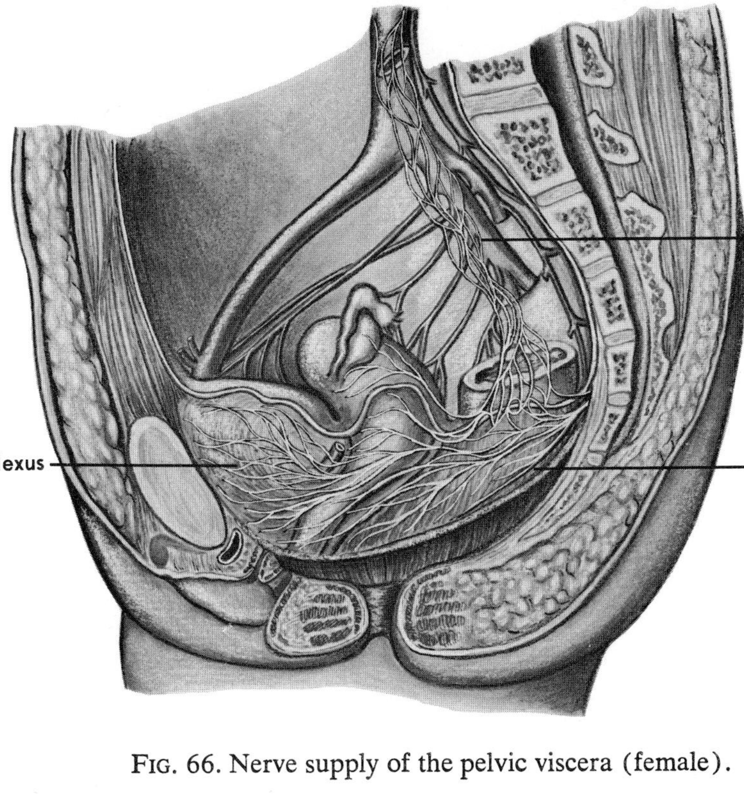

FIG. 66. Nerve supply of the pelvic viscera (female).

Preganglionic fibers of the sacral portion of the parasympathetic pathway arise from the intermediolateral cell column of the gray matter in the 2nd, the 3rd and the 4th sacral segments of the spinal cord and pass by way of 3 to 6 white communicating rami, emerging as the pelvic nerve or the nervi erigentes. These pelvic and splanchnic nerves continue to form the pelvic plexus of Frankenhauser, on each side of the hypogastric plexus, at the site of the prostate gland, the base of the urinary bladder, and the rectum. Branches are distributed from here to the rest of the transverse, descending and the pelvic portions of the colon. Other branches of the plexus communicate with the hypogastric plexus of the sympathetic system, which is thus distributed with the middle hemorrhoidal artery to the rectum, and with the vessels supplying the urinary bladder and the genitalia.

These preganglionic parasympathetic fibers synapse in the terminal ganglia located in the wall of the bowel. They form Meissner's submucosal and Auerbach's intermuscular plexuses. These 2 intramural plexuses intercommunicate with one another. The submucosal plexus is distributed mainly to the glands of the muscularis mucosae, ramifying in the submucosa, between and around the glands. Primary, secondary and even tertiary ramifications of the myenteric plexus have been described as they are distributed to the muscle coats. The number of myenteric plexuses progressively increases as one proceeds distally along the colon, and in the rectum they are almost as abundant as in the pylorus.

Postganglionic fibers are also demonstrable in the subepithelial plexus of the rectum.

The parasympathetic supply of the internal anal sphincter is more or less the same as that of the rectum, being distributed with the inferior hemorrhoidal artery (together with the sympathetics), from the internal pudendal.

Visceral Sensory System

Painful visceral sensations are aroused by stimuli different from those that cause somatic pain. The latter may be mechanical, thermal, chemical or electric, while the former include distention, violent and spastic smooth muscle contraction and deficient blood supply. Owing to the presence of central connections, this visceral sensory system is not considered to be a part of the autonomic system. Essentially, it is a reflex autonomic arc.

The precise localization of these autonomic viscerosensory conduction pathways is not definitely known. The peripheral nerve processes of the visceral afferent nerve fibers from the visceroreceptor nerve endings in the epithelial nerve plexuses of the colon pass through the sympathetic ganglia without synapse. Through the white rami communicantes they enter the spinal nerve at the 11th and the 12th thoracic and the 1st lumbar. The ganglia are located in the dorsal root ganglia of the spinal nerve, together with the somatic afferent fibers. The central process of the nerve passes out of the dorsolateral portion of the gray matter of the spinal cord after sending short ascending and descending branches to the dorsolateral funiculus of the white matter. The synapse occurs in the dorsolateral horn and with an intercalated neuron in the intermediolateral column.

Viscerosensory impulses from the rectum are conducted through the pelvic nerves (2nd and 3rd sacral) to the spinal cord.

From the intermediolateral column,

preganglionic visceral efferent fibers leave through the ventral nerve root, the spinal nerve and the white rami communicantes and traverse the sympathetic trunk. A synapse is first formed in the collateral sympathetic ganglia (which differentiates it from the somatic reflex arc); from thence the postganglionic fibers reach the walls of the colon. In other instances a synapse may be formed in the ganglia, passing through the gray rami communicantes and the spinal nerve into the blood vessels of the colon.

Autonomic Supply of the Anal Canal and the Perianal Skin

Sympathetic fibers of the anal skin and part of the parietal sympathetics (in contrast with the visceral sympathetics of the colon and the rectum), arise chiefly from the sacral and the coccygeal ganglia. They are distributed to the glands and the vessels of the perianal skin.

The parasympathetic supply of the anal canal probably is a continuation of the intermuscular plexus of Auerbach, as a plexus of the conjoined longitudinal muscle band that reaches the perianal skin.

Meissner's submucosal plexus probably communicates and is continuous with the subepithelial plexus of the perianal skin to reach the sweat, the sebaceous and the apocrine glands of the perianal skin. Interestingly enough, a bulbous ganglionic enlargement has been described in the anal papilla as it lies close to the base of the column of Morgagni.

The terminal distribution of the nerves of the anorectal sphincter has been shown to present free anastomosis between the terminal arborization and ganglion cells, containing sensory, motor and sympathetic end plates.

Cerebrospinal Nerve Supply of the Anal Canal and the Perianal Skin

In addition to its autonomic nerve supply, the anal canal and the perianal skin receive branches from the cerebrospinal nervous system for somatic motor and somatic sensory function. These nerves are derived mainly from the 3rd, the 4th and the 5th sacral segments and from filaments of the coccygeal nerves. These are distributed by the peripheral nerves which reach the anal musculature through the anoderm and the perianal skin.

The peripheral nerves include the inferior hemorrhoidal nerve, the anterior sphincterian nerve, and the perineal branches of the 4th sacral and the coccygeal nerves. The inferior hemorrhoidal nerve is a branch of the internal pudendal nerve and generally follows the distribution of the inferior hemorrhoidal artery with which it forms the inferior neurovascular stalk. Usually, it sends muscular branches to the 3 divisions of the external sphincter, together with the lateral sphincteric branches of the inferior hemorrhoidal artery. Aside from the terminal distribution in the muscle, terminals are sent also to the perianal skin and the anorectal junction.

The anterior sphincterian nerve of Tuttle is distributed with the artery of the same name (the anterior sphincterian artery or the transverse perineal branch of the inferior hemorrhoidal artery). It sends branches to the anterolateral aspect of the external sphincter and the subjacent portion of the perianal skin.

The perineal branch of the 4th sacral is essentially a cutaneous nerve and innervates the posterior phase of the anal triangle.

Numerous twigs arising from the coc-

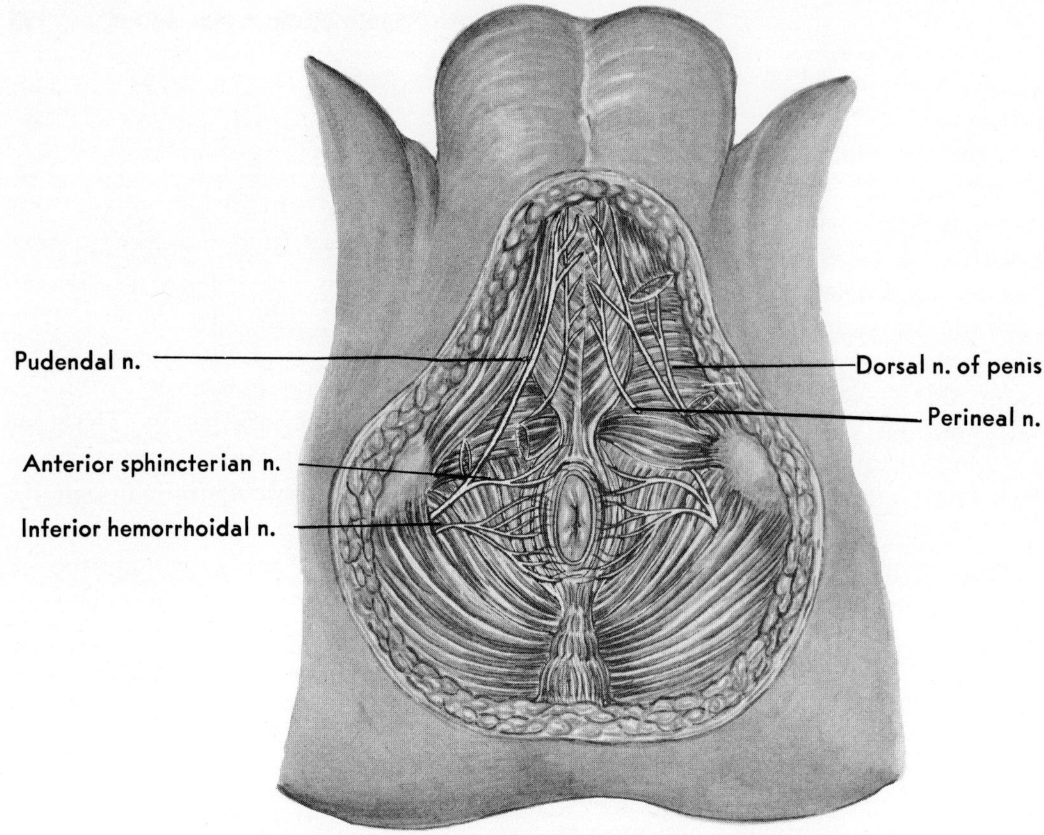
Pudendal n.
Dorsal n. of penis
Perineal n.
Anterior sphincterian n.
Inferior hemorrhoidal n.

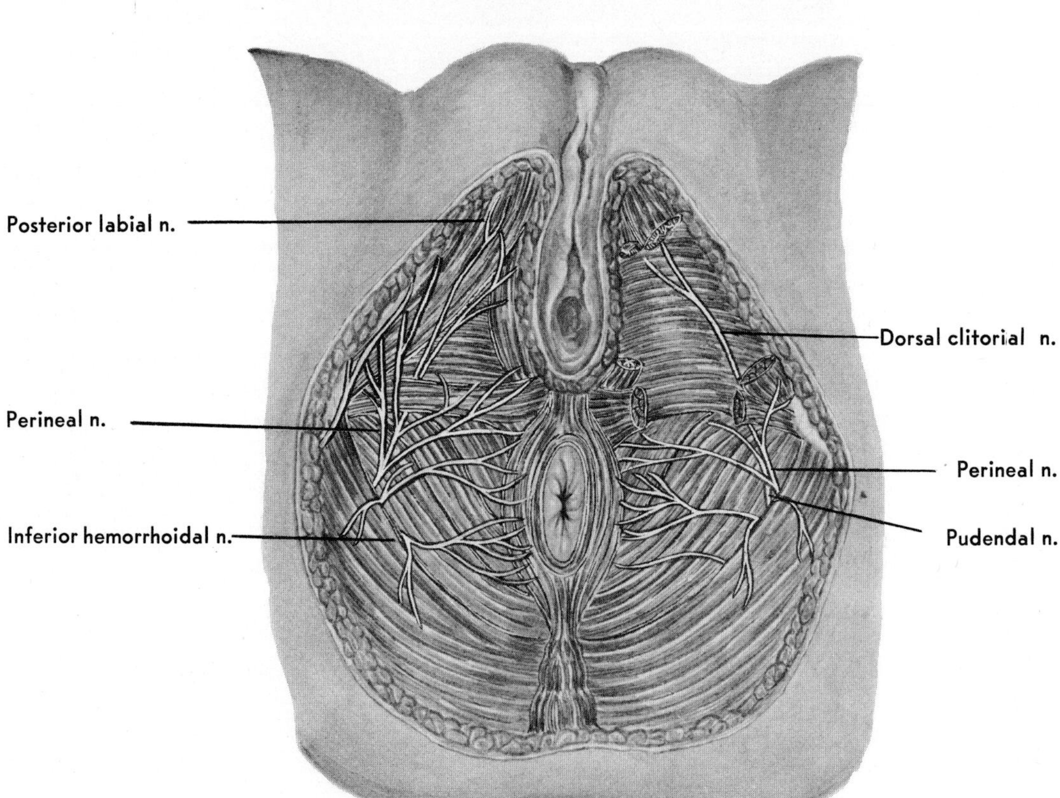
Posterior labial n.
Dorsal clitorial n.
Perineal n.
Perineal n.
Inferior hemorrhoidal n.
Pudendal n.

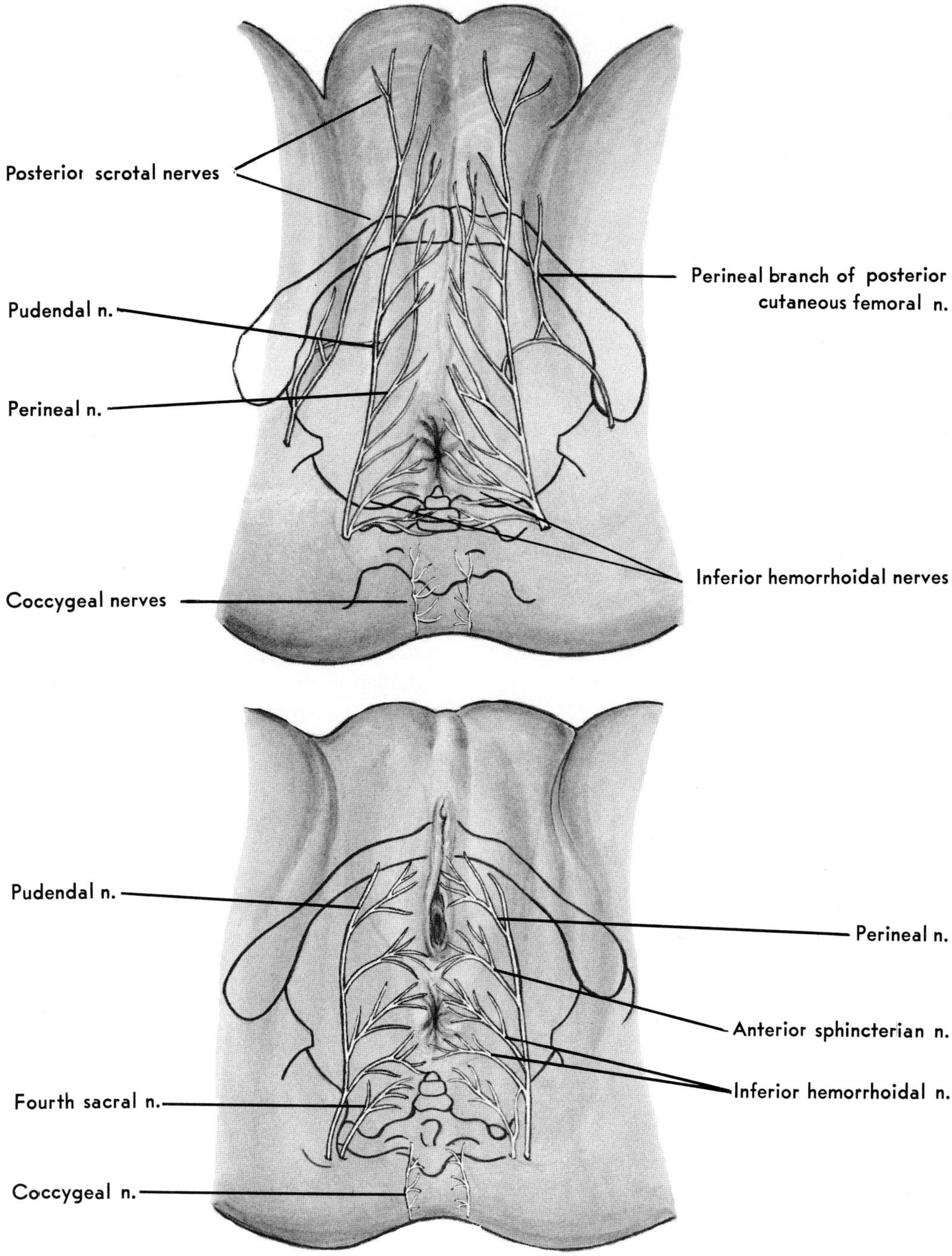

FIG. 67 (*Facing page, top*). Nerve supply of the male perineum.
FIG. 68 (*Facing page, bottom*). Nerve supply of the female perineum.
FIG. 69 (*Above*). Distribution and location of sensory nerves of the anal region (male and female).

cygeal nerves are disposed in two sets: an anterior and a posterior. The anterior set supplies the anococcygeal area alone with the anococcygeal branch of the inferior hemorrhoidal artery. A large terminal filament is called the posterior sphincter nerve. The posterior branch ramifies over the coccygeal skin and inosculates with the dorsal branch of the sacral nerve.

The anoderm and the perianal skin are abundantly supplied with nerves and therefore are unusually sensitive. The nerves supplying the anal skin are the same as those supplying the anorectal sphincter. Thus severe spasm follows irritation of the nerve endings in the anal skin. This is best demonstrated clinically in the case of anal fissures or intra-anal ulcers.

By contrast, the absense of cerebrospinal somatic sensory nerves in the rectum prevents large, ulcerating and infected carcinomas of the ampulla from evoking pain as long as the lesion is confined to the rectal wall and has not invaded the anal skin or the nearby nerve plexuses.

The internal pudendal nerve also supplies the compressor urethra, while the 3rd and the 4th sacral nerves supply the urinary bladder, the prostate and the vagina. All these nerves arise from the lumbar enlargement of the cord, from which also arise the small and the great sciatic nerves.

Surgical Considerations

Following various procedures of proctocolectomy, be it transabdominal or combined abdominoperineal resection or excision, bladder dysfunction or sexual impotence are complications in a certain percentage of patients and are due to injury or section of the hypogastric and the sacropelvic nerves, which results in vesical atonia, and section of the nervi erigenti, which results in sexual impotence. Therefore, it is important to enter the proper cleavage plane when performing blunt dissection of the rectum from the hollow of the sacrum. For nonmalignant conditions, injury to the nervi erigentes can be prevented by dissecting close to the rectum. However, in no instance should a compromise of the dissection be made for cancer operations, especially of low rectal or anal lesions, to preserve the nerve.

Vesical dysfunction is usually temporary, and bladder distention is prevented postoperatively by leaving a Foley catheter for 5 days. Occasionally, the catheter must be reinserted if the residual urine is more than 60 to 100 cc. Intrinsic nerves of the bladder have been demonstrated, which accounts for re-establishment of bladder function following injury to the hypogastric plexus and the sacropelvic nerves, although such re-establishment of function may require as long as 5 months of catheter drainage.

Following abdominoperineal excision (Miles), about 95 per cent of male patients become sexually impotent. In the experience of the senior author (H.E.B.) 12.2 per cent of patients following pull-through operations have some sexual dysfunction: 7.7 per cent were impotent, and 4.5 per cent achieved erections but no ejaculation. When these operations are performed in the younger age group for nonmalignant conditions, typical of which is ulcerative colitis, it is advisable to warn them of such a complication, although a meticulous dissection in the cleavage planes close to the rectum avoids this misfortune. In our entire series in whom colectomy was performed for ulcerative colitis, only one instance of impotence was experienced.

Control of feces is normal after anterior resection except in patients with low anastomoses, who may experience rectal tenesmus and urgency for variable periods of time, although ordinarily these symptoms recede spontaneously. On the other hand, combined abdominoperineal proctosigmoidectomy with preservation of the anal sphincters has been criticized uninhibitedly from the standpoint of fecal continence. In the senior author's experience, all are continent, although approximately 41 per cent use irrigations to initiate defecation. Of 704 patients operated upon for cancer, only 2, or .03 per cent use a perineal pad. Admittedly, others who have performed similar procedures have obtained far less success and therefore have been vehemently and staunchly critical of the procedure, in spite of comparable long-term survival rates of 5, 10 and 15 years.

From the surgical point of view, the rectal mucosa is regarded as insensitive, although it is possessed of visceral sensory fibers which are conveyed through the parasympathetic and the hypogastric nerves. Those conveyed through the former are the normal sensation of physiologic distention, and those conveyed through the latter are pain sensations resulting from overdistention or excessive spasm. Hence, patients often feel a sensation of distention following submucous injection of hemorrhoids or during proctosigmoidoscopy. There may also be an overlapping of the peripheral nerve supply at the anorectal line, extending superiorly for 1 to 1½ cm. Hence, incision and drainage of a low submucous abscess may require anesthesia.

The anal canal is supplied by the inferior hemorrhoidal nerve, a branch of the internal pudendal nerve. Through the latter, reflex dysfunctions of the adjacent organs of the genitourinary systems of anorectal origin are set up. Hence, the presence of a painful anal lesion, such as fissure, thrombosed hemorrhoids, surgical wounds following operations or cryptitis, may cause urinary retention, dysuria, dysmenorrhea, dyspareunia, lumbosacral pain, pain along the iliac crest and the posterior aspect of the thigh, and locally there is associated marked spasm of the anal sphincters.

Chapter 3

Physiology of Colon and Rectum

COMPARATIVE PHYSIOLOGY

The colon has not been proved to be essential to a normally active life, much less to a comfortable existence. Man's omniverous eating habits have evolved for him a long segmented colon which combines the essential features of the absorptive and the digestive types found in herbivores with the storage and the excretory types found in flesh-eating carnivores. The former have a long colon with a large cecum, suitable for bacterial digestion. The latter have a short colon and a rudimentary cecum adaptable for digestive fermentation.

The right colon develops from the midgut; it is supplied by the superior mesenteric artery, innervated by the vagus and is concerned with the absorption and the dehydration of the digested food. The left colon develops from the hindgut; it is supplied by the inferior mesenteric artery, innervated by the sacral parasympathetics and is concerned with the storage and the expulsion of the stool.

SECRETION

The normal secretion of the colon is alkaline. It consists of lubricating mucus derived from the goblet cells in the crypts of Lieberkühn, mixed with tissue detritus, and the salts of calcium, magnesium, and all heavy metals that may be present in the body. The amount of mucus increases as one proceeds distally, until in the rectum there may be many more goblet cells than in the more proximal portions.

BACTERIA

Intestinal bacteria abound in the terminal ileum, the cecum and the right hemicolon, where the alkaline conditions apparently are ideal for the putrefactive processes. Bacterial bodies constitute about 9 per cent of the stool. The nature of the bacterial flora is affected by diet. The bacterial population of the normal stool consists of coliform bacilli (70%), bacteroides group (20%), streptococci (8%), spore bearers (0.001%) and a heterogenous group (2%) composed of yeasts, proteus, pseudomonas and lactobacilli and staphylococci. It is this heterogenous group that proliferates very rapidly and flourishes after the rest of the colonic micro-organisms are killed by antibiotics. After the first feeding of the newborn, these organisms may be demonstrated or detected in the stool.

Between the predominating coliform bacilli and the aerobacter group are numerous organisms that belong to the paracolon group. These intermediate organisms have their own distinguishing fermentative characteristics.

Higher micro-organisms besides yeasts, like protozoa and spirochetes, may also be found in small numbers. The latter apparently have migrated from the mouth.

The spore-bearers may be either aerobes or anaerobes, and both pathogenic and nonpathogenic. It is probable that they represent the smallest group of micro-organisms in the colon.

These micro-organisms digest cellulose and take part in the synthesis and the absorption of vitamins B and K_2. Among the factors of the vitamin B complex affected are thiamine, riboflavin, nicotinic acid, cyanocoabalamine, folic acid, biotin, pantothenic acid and pyridoxine. They also produce gas in the intestine, flavored by the products of putrefaction. Hence, when antibiotics are administered, they compete with the enzyme system needed for the metabolic processes of the bacteria. The coliform and other predominating organisms die, but later on, one minority group may flourish, suddenly becoming pathogenic and invading the tissue of the host. When these organisms die, the stool and the flatus become odorless and less in amount; after prolonged antibiotic administration, faulty vitamin synthesis and absorption occurs, leading to hypovitaminosis. Thus, there may result metabolic, muscular and nervous dysfunction, macrocytic anemia and a hemorrhagic diathesis.

STOOL

The stool represents an aggregate of secretion (mucus and bile pigments) and the products of the intestinal tract (cholesterol, purine bases, salts of calcium, iron and magnesium), tissue detritus (epithelial cells), bacterial bodies, residue of digested as well as indigestible food particles and minute quantities of vitamins. The stool normally is evacuated as cylindrical segments 10 to 20 cm. long and 2 to 4 cm. in diameter, with an average total weight of 100 to 200 Gm., of which 25 Gm. are solid, and equivalent to 70 to 140 calories.

A protein-rich diet produces a dark-brown or yellow, offensive, hard, almost scybalous stool with many gram-positive organisms. A carbohydrate diet produces a greenish-brown, foul, mushy, soft, semifluid, acidic stool with many gram-negative organisms. As a rule, the normal stool has a brown shade due to the presence of stercobilin and urobilin. The color depends upon the diet and is altered by certain medications.

Normally, the stool is alkaline, pH 6.9 to 7.7, the degree of alkalinity being in direct proportion to its length of stay in the colon. Thus, loose stools are generally acidic and therefore irritating to the perianal skin.

FLATUS

Colonic flatus results from bacterial activity in the proximal colon and consists of methane (25%), hydrogen sulfide (5%), nitrogen (60%), and carbon dioxide (10%). As much as a liter of flatus may be expelled in 24 hours. The average single discharge of gas measures 100 cc., although the amount usually varies from 50 to 300 cc. The odor varies with the diet and is influenced by the different gases that enter into its composition.

Occasionally, excessive formation of hydrogen sulfide will cause sulfhemoglobinemia, which in excessive amount may cause cyanosis. This is called enterogenous cyanosis, as distinguished from sulfhemoglobinemia secondary to drugs like phenacetin.

Normally, about 750 to 2,500 cc. of gas is found within the colon. This gas comes from swallowed air (500 to 1,000 cc.) or as a result of bacterial activity which causes diffusion from the blood stream. Thus air swallowed with food, drink, or during phonation and respiration is the largest source of intestinal gas. The oldtime injunction to maintain starvation and silence postoperatively has some physiologic basis as far as the origin of intestinal gas is concerned.

Intestinal gas aids in inducing peristalsis by distending the bowel slightly, just to the point of initiating a peristaltic wave. The more motile a bowel is, the more gas it contains. Peristalsis, together with the movements of the normal amounts of gas inside the bowel, is responsible for the fine crackling sounds normally detected during abdominal auscultation. Such sounds are absent during paralytic ileus, because despite the presence of gas and fluid, there is no peristaltic wave. In cases of mechanical obstruction, these sounds become accentuated, owing to the vigorous peristalsis that tries to force the trapped gas and intestinal secretions beyond the obstruction. In obstruction, the sounds vary from low-pitched cracklings to high-pitched tinkles. When rapid peristalsis occurs in a colon distended with fluid, there will be audible borborygmi.

Gas in the bowel may be expelled as a belch, as colonic flatus or even be absorbed back into the circulation. Vigorous inhalation of almost pure oxygen has been proved to displace the nitrogen component of the intestinal gas. Gaseous distention naturally follows inadequate absorption and expulsion of gases; it may mean more swallowed air but not necessarily more gas formation.

Excessive gas in the colon results in the stretching of the walls of the bowel with its contained nerve plexus and is therefore interpreted as pain. Owing to the distended bowel, there is insufficient peristalsis, with increasing intra-abdominal pressure and decrease in pulmonary ventilation, reducing venous return and cardiac filling. This finally leads to reduction of pulmonary gas exchange and ultimately reduced blood flow from the lungs. Thus, a vicious cycle is set up.

Should such gas collections occur postoperatively, they may endanger the integrity of the suture line; embarrass respiration, causing atelectasis; embarrass circulation, delaying regenerative processes and encouraging thrombosis. The vicious cycle continues with distention leading to compression of the intramural vessels, causing stagnation of absorption, thus resulting further in increased gas collection. Furthermore, the decreased cardiorespiratory efficiency also reduces the absorption of intestinal gases.

Intestinal gases, like any other gas, follow Boyle's law, so that at ½ atmospheric pressure, the volume of gas in the bowel is double that present at 1 atmospheric pressure. Thus, in ascent in airplanes, there is an increased amount of intestinal gas, but because the tone and the viability of the bowel wall are maintained, gas absorption and expulsion are not hindered. Above 14,000 feet, however, the rate of the expansion of gas exceeds that of its expulsion and absorption; therefore, gas distention occurs. A rapid ascent of about 1,100 feet per minute will trap the gas in the bowel segments and cause gas pains.

MOTILITY AND PERISTALSIS

The muscular coat of the bowel behaves like smooth muscle anywhere. Spontaneous muscular activity called motility is characteristic of the bowel. This activity is controlled by numerous neurohumoral and possibly prophysiologic mechanisms. Normally, the walls are in a state of tone, and distention beyond a certain threshold value provides further stimuli for increased muscular activity, although distally the colon is known to be able to adapt itself to the enlarging fecal mass. Peristalsis refers to the activity that results in the propulsion or forward movement of the intestinal contents. Rhythm denotes a constant rate and pressure among the contraction waves so that they more or less conform to a definite pattern.

Peristalsis always progresses toward the anal opening, probably due to some inherent nervous mechanism in the bowel, which is responsible for the co-ordination of anatomically indefinable but physiologically demonstrable segments. While peristalsis may be influenced by the central nervous system, paralysis of the nerve cells does not abolish this muscular activity. A decreasing intracolonic pressure gradient has been thought to be principally responsible for the forward movement of peristalsis.

The basic wave patterns in the human gastrointestinal tract have been classified into 4 types.

1. Type 1—small, simple nonpropulsive waves.
2. Type 2—large, simple mixing waves which appear to be magnified Type 1 and probably are responsible for the haustrations.
3. Type 3—complex waves, representing either Type 1 or Type 2 superimposed upon a change in tonus, which are neither propulsive nor mixing.
4. Type 4—large smooth propulsive waves usually seen just before defecation.

Both proximal and distal segments of the colon follow the same basic configuration of the wave patterns. However, in the distal segment waves of all types are usually of lower tone and have less intraluminal pressure variation. This decrease in pressure values possibly accounts for the forward movement of the intestinal contents.

The rate of the progress of intestinal peristalsis is governed by numerous factors, both intrinsic and extrinsic, neurohumoral and biophysiologic. Among the intrinsic factors are changes in the chemistry and the acid-base equilibrium of the body fluids. The extrinsic factors include the act of swallowing and the presence of fullness, exercise, and intake of drugs.

Defecation refers to the neurophysical act of the expulsion of the stool, while continence implies voluntary control over the process until the movement is more convenient or the setting more suitable. Constipation is the undue delay in the passage of stool, resulting in the evacuation of dehydrated lumps of feces, while the undue haste in the passage of feces through the gut is called diarrhea. The frequency and the regularity of bowel movement is a purely individual characteristic, under the control of habit and education. While a daily bowel movement is universally accepted as normal and desirable, that regularity which an individual has established for himself should be considered as normal for that particular individual. Constipation can result from decreased bulk of stool, the presence of obstructive hypertonicity with resulting spasm of the wall, and the impairment of reflexes. Diarrhea will follow increased bulk of stool, increased tone of the small bowel, inflammation and irritability of the bowel wall, and an unusually sensitive nervous system.

The reflex of defecation is mediated through a reflex arc, with the basic components of receptor, afferent fiber, nerve center, efferent fiber and effector. The distal colon and the rectum normally are empty except when defecation is about to begin. The distal colon fills up as a result of mass movement, a massive peristaltic rush initiated by a habitual act as getting out of bed, drinking a cup of coffee, smoking a cigarette, and the passage of food through the pylorus. The fecal mass is shoved through the distal colon and the rectum into the anorectal region where the receptors are located. This gives the urge to defecate which is felt as heaviness deep-seated in the perineum or low in the sacrococcygeal area.

These impulses are carried by afferents, through the sacral parasympathetic to the spinal cord. The spinal center for defecation is located in the conus medullaris opposite the first lumbar vertebra.

High cerebral centers may modify the response of the effectors, although they have no absolute control over the act. The supervisory function exercised by the cortical centers varies, depending largely upon the previous training and experience of the individual, and is conditioned mainly by what has been vaguely termed education, breeding and civilization. As a rule, central inhibition postpones the act; but occasionally, despite violent cerebral resistance, the act can be accomplished. Impulses are then sent to the cord through the sympathetics to increase the tone of the sphincters and to relax the sigmoid. Central inhibition is followed by a retroperistaltic wave that retrojects the stool back into the sigmoid and the descending colon. The distention of the distal colon by the retrojected mass is referred to as visceral sensation in the corresponding somite. This may be felt as a heaviness in the left iliac region or in the lower abdomen. Thus when conscious levels disregard the urge to defecate, the threshold value of the stimulus is raised, and the distal colon adapts itself to the enlarging fecal mass.

Once cortical consent is given, the active phase of defecation begins. The longitudinal muscle bands of the rectum, which are fixed at the rectococcygeus muscles, are shortened, and the nerve impulses are mediated through the sacral parasympathetics over the sacral plexus to the related muscles. The internal anal sphincter relaxes, and the fecal mass passes, and the contiguous external sphincter relaxes also. The levator ani muscle contracts to stretch the relaxed anal sphincters, and pulls above the fecal mass, widening the anorectal angle at the same time to allow the fecal mass to go through. The transit of the fecal mass is facilitated by the increased intra-abdominal pressure brought about by the contraction of the diaphragm at the end of expiration, a synchronous closure of the glottis, contraction of the muscles of the anterior abdominal wall, aided by the pressure of the thigh muscles against the abdomen. The increased intra-abdominal pressure compresses the sigmoid and forces the feces down the rectum.

When the anorectal sphincters contract and the voluntary muscles of the abdominal wall relax, a segment of the stool is pinched off, and the latter falls off by its own weight. The walls of the anal canal are once more in apposition, and the corrugator cutis ani clears out any particle of stool left on the perianal skin. In animals this function of the corrugators is well preserved. In man the corrugator is part of the longitudinal muscle band of the rectum, and when the latter contracts the corrugations are deepened. When the muscle relaxes after defecation, the corrugations become shallower, thus throwing off any particle that may have become lodged with the passage of the previous fecal lump. The act may be finished, or another active phase of defecation begins. Should the act be finished, then any unexpelled stool is retrojected into the sigmoid. Voluntary control or re-enforcement of the act is apparently a matter of exigency, modified by the habit, training and psychologic pattern of the individual.

The normal intracolonic pressure is 20 mm. Hg. At 40 to 50 mm. Hg the defecation reflex is void, and the pressure may be increased to 100 to 200 mm. Hg upon straining. This increased intra-abdominal pressure is transmitted to the vascular system, the cerebrospinal spaces and the thoracic cavity.

The parasympathetics increase the bowel tone and relax the sphincters, while the sympathetics decrease the bowel tone and contract the sphincters. The former are called the emptying nerves, while the latter are referred to as the filling nerves. Therefore, stimulation of the parasympathetics will induce evacuation, while stimulation of the sympathetics will cause an inhibition of the activity and closure of the sphincters.

After section of the spinal cord, or in the untrained newborn, the discharge of stool into the rectum and the anorectal line will cause stimulation of the pelvic nerves, which then relax the sphincter. This is called the automatic rectum.

The external anal sphincter is composed of striated muscle; it does not degenerate, despite section of the internal pudendal nerve. The functional ability probably is retained by the intra-epithelial neuronlike argyrophile cells found in the anal canal.

The destruction of the spinal cord will abolish the tonic contraction of the sphincter. Stimulation or inhibition of the sphincters could be initiated by a peripheral stimulus as by stroking, or applying heat to the perineum, etc., or by an emotional factor, as fear. Section of the pelvic nerves will cause relaxation of the walls of the distal colon, and section of the cord above the sacral segment will similarly cause relaxation.

Distention of the rectum causes reflex hypertension which stretches the pain-sensitive intracranial arteries, probably explaining the headaches that accompany constipation. Since constipation may be due to deficient bile flow; this is probably the explanation of the oldtime biliousness or the irritability of the individual with liver disease.

Very little digestion takes place in the colon. Whatever digestion does occur is due to continued action of enteric ferments upon the undigested food, as both are passed as chyme through the ileocecal valve. Absorption in the colon usually involves the water, the digesta and the mucus of colonic secretion.

Various sphincters have been described in the colorectoanal tract. They include:

1. Ileocolic sphincter of Varolius, Bauhinus, Tulpius or Vidulius, possesses a definite sphincter action with a definite muscle demonstrable.

2. Colicocecal sphincter of Busi, demonstrable by roentgenograms, shows increased longitudinal and circular muscle, marked externally by a cecal furrow.

3. Ascending colic sphincter of Hirsch, located 2½ in. above the ileocecal sphincter, where the lumen narrows and the walls thicken.

4. Transverse colic sphincter of Cannon, located between the hepatic flexure and the midtransverse colon. It represents a radiologic landmark and may well be an anatomophysiologic point.

5. Transverse colic sphincter of Payr and Strauss, located on the left half of the transverse colon, near the splenic flexure but without demonstrable increase in the circular muscle.

6. Colicosigmoid sphincter of Busi, where the descending colon and the sigmoid meet.

7. Rectosigmoid sphincter of Moutier and O'Beirne, demonstrable proctoscopically and radiologically.

8. Internal anal sphincter, the thickening of the circular muscle at the lower end of the rectum.

9. External anal sphincter, which has been divided into 3 components: subcutaneous, superficial and deep portions.

Bibliography

EMBRYOLOGY

Arey, L. B.: Developmental Anatomy, ed. 5, Philadelphia, Saunders, 1946.

Bacon, H. E.: Histology and embryology of the anorectal line, Tr. Am. Proct. Soc. *33*:144, 1932.

Bacon, H. E., Ross, S. T., and Recio, P. M.: Proctology, Philadelphia, Lippincott, 1956.

Barrett, C. W.: A study of the anatomy, embryology, and function of the anus in relation to the caudal wall, J. Nat. Proct. A. *19*:15, 1946.

——: Anatomy and embryology of the anus in relation to the pelvic floor, J. Internat. Coll. Surgeons *10*:308, 1947.

Bodenhammer, W. M.: Practical Observations on Some of the Diseases of the Rectum, Anus, and Contiguous Structures, Cincinnati, Sparhawk, 1874.

Boyden, E. A.: Early development of the cloaca in ostrich embryos with special reference to the reduction of the caudal intestine, Anat. Rec. *24*:211, 1922.

——: The development of the cloaca of birds, with special reference to the origin of the bursa of Fabricus, the formation of a urodeal sinus and the regular occurrence of a cloacal fenestra, Am. J. Anat. *30*:163, 1922.

Dott, N.: Anomalies of intestinal rotation: their embryology and surgical aspects with report of 5 cases, Brit. J. Surg. *11*:251, 1923.

Gerrish, F. H.: Textbook of Anatomy, Philadelphia, Lea Bros., 1899.

Grinvaslky, H. T., and Helwig, E. B.: Carcinoma of the anorectal junction, Cancer *9*: 480, 1956.

Gross, R. E.: The Surgery of Infancy and Childhood, Philadelphia, Saunders, 1953.

Hamilton, W. J., Boyd, J. D., and Mossman, H. W.: Human Embryology, Baltimore, Williams & Wilkins, 1945.

Hermann, G.: Sur la structure et le développement de la muqueuse anale, J. Lancet et physiol. *16*:434, 1880.

Johnson, F.: The development of the rectum in the human embryo, Am. J. Anat. *16*:1, 1914.

Keibel, F., and Mall, F.: A Manual of Human Embryology, vol. 1, Philadelphia, Lippincott, 1910.

Keith, H.: Human Embryology, ed. 4, London, E. Arnold, 1921.

Ladd, W. E., and Gross, R. E.: Surgical treatment of duplications of the alimentary tract: enterogenous cysts, enteric cysts, or ileum duplex, Surg., Gynec. & Obst. *70*:295, 1940.

Mall, F.: Development of the human intestine and its position in the adult, Bull. Johns Hopkins Hosp. *20*:197, 1889.

Patten, B. M.: Human Embryology, Philadelphia, Blakiston, 1947.

Power, R. M.: Embryological development of the levator ani muscle, Am. J. Obst. & Gynec. *55*:367, 1948.

Tench, E. M.: Development of the anus in the human embryo, Am. J. Anat. *59*:333, 1936.

COLON

Anson, B. J.: Atlas of Human Anatomy, Philadelphia, Saunders, 1950.

Bacon, H. E., Ross, S. T., and Recio, P. M.: Proctology, Philadelphia, Lippincott, 1956.

Berry, R. J.: The Anatomy of the Cecum, Anatomischer Anzeiger, v. 10, 1886.

——: Cecal Folds and Fossae and the Topographical Anatomy of the Vermiform Appendix, Edinburgh, W. J. Clay, 1897.

Corning, H. K.: Lehrbuch der topographischen Anatomie, ed. 8, Munich, Bergmann, 1919.

Cruveilhier, J.: Traité d'anatomie pathologique générale, vol. 3, Paris, Baillière, 1849.

Cunningham, D. J.: Textbook of Anatomy, ed. 5, New York, Wm. Wood & Co., 1921.

Davis, G. G.: Applied Anatomy, ed. 9, Philadelphia, Lippincott, 1934.

Goodsall, D. H., and Miles, W. E.: Diseases of the Anus and Rectum, London, Longmans, 1900.

Gorsh, R. V.: Proctologic Anatomy, Baltimore, Williams & Wilkins, 1946.

Grant, J. C.: A Method of Anatomy, ed. 3, Baltimore, Williams & Wilkins, 1944.

Gross, R. E.: The Surgery of Infancy and Childhood, Philadelphia, Saunders, 1953.

Jackman, R. J.: The importance and technique of proctoscopy, Dis. Colon & Rectum *2*:139, 1959.

Laimer, E.: Zur Anatomie des Mastdarmes, Med. Jahrb. Wien *49*:49, 1884.

Last, R.: Anatomy: Regional and Applied, Boston, Little, 1954.

Lewis, W.: Gray's Anatomy, ed. 24, Philadelphia, Lea & Febiger, 1942.

Lieberkuhn, J.: Dissertatio anatomica-physiologica de fabrica et Actione villirun intestinorum tenium hominis, Leyden, 1745.

Matthews, J.: Treatise on Diseases of the Rectum, Anus, and Sigmoid Flexure, New York, Appleton, 1892.

McGregor, A. L.: A Synopsis of Surgical Anatomy, ed. 5, Baltimore, Williams & Wilkins, 1946.

Merkel, F.: Handbuch der topographischen Anatomie, Braunschweig, vol. 3, 1903.

Miles, W. E.: Cancer of the Rectum, London, Harrison, 1926.

Monks, G.: Intestinal localization: a review of certain studies in the surgical anatomy of the small intestine and its mesentery, Surg., Gynec. & Obst. *49*:213, 1929.

Morton, D. J.: Human Anatomy, New York, Columbia Press, 1934.

Paitre, F., Giraud, D., and Dupret, S.: Pratique Anatomo-Chirurgicale, Paris, Doin, 1935.

Pennington, J. R.: A Treatise on Diseases of the Anus, Rectum, and Pelvic Colon, Philadelphia, Blakiston, 1923.

Piersol, G.: Human Anatomy, ed. 6, Philadelphia, Lippincott, 1930.

Poirier P. and Charpy A.: Traité d'anatomie humaine Paris Masson 1889.

Quains, J.: Elements of Anatomy, ed. 10, London, Longmans, 1921.

Sappey, M.: Traité d'anatomie humaine, anatomie descriptive, ed. 4, vol. 4, Paris, Delahaye et Lecrosnier, 1889.

Schaeffer, J.: Morris' Human Anatomy, ed. 10, Philadelphia, Blakiston, 1951.

Spalteholz, W. A.: Atlas of Human Anatomy, ed. 14, vol. 3, Leipzig, Hirzel, 1914.

Swenson, O., Rheinlander, H. F., and Diamond, I.: Hirschprung's disease: a new concept of etiology, New England J. Med. *241*: 551, 1949.

Testut, L.: Traité d'anatomie humaine, ed. 5, Paris, Doin, 1904.

——: Traité d'anatomie topographique, Paris, Doin, 1906.

Testut, L., and Jacob, O.: Traité d'anatomie topographique, vol. 2, Paris, Doin, 1906.

Thorek: P.: Anatomy in Surgery, Philadelphia, Lippincott, 1951.

Uhlenhuth, E.: Sobatta's Atlas of Descriptive Anatomy, English ed. 6, Philadelphia, Saunders, 1911.

Wood-Jones, F.: Buchanan's Manual of Anatomy, ed. 7, Baltimore, Williams & Wilkins, 1946.

RECTUM AND ANAL CANAL

Bacon, H. E.: Histology and embryology of the anorectal line, Tr. Am. Proct. Soc. *33*:144, 1932.

Bacon, H. E., Ross, S. T., and Recio, P. M.: Proctology, Philadelphia, Lippincott, 1956.

Beraud, M.: Manner of termination of the longitudinal fibers of the rectum, Compt. rend. Soc. biol. *4*:163, 1857.

Courtney, H.: Anatomy of the pelvic diaphragm and anorectal musculature as related to sphincter preservation in anorectal surgery, Tr. Am. Proct. Soc. *48*:155, 1949.

Dunphy, J.: Surgical anatomy of the anal canal, Arch. Surg. *57*:791, 1948.

Fine, J., and Lawes, C.: Muscle fibers of the anal submucosa with special reference to the pecten band, Brit. J. Surg. *27*:723, 1940.

Gay, A.: Die Circumanaldrusen des Menschen, Sitz. ber. d. Kais. Akad. d. Wiss. *63*:329, 1871.

Glisson, F.: Traité sur l'anatomie, vol. 4, Paris, 1637.

Hermann, G., and Desfosses, L.: Sur la muqueuse de la région cloacle du rectum, Compt. rend Acad. sc. *90*:130, 1880.

Hibshman, H.: Personal communication on intersphincteric line.

Hill, M. R., Shyrock, E. H., and ReBell, F. G.: The role of anal glands in pathogenesis of anorectal disease, J.A.M.A. *121*:742, 1943.

Hiller, R. I.: Anal anatomy with special reference to the white line of Hilton and the pecten of Stroud, Ann. Surg. *102*:81, 1935.

Hilton, J.: Rest and Pain, London, Bell, 1876.

Holl, M.: Anatomie, ed. 4, part 2, vol. 7, Jena, Fischer, 1897.

Horner, W. A.: A Treatise on Special and General Anatomy, vol. 2, Philadelphia, Carey, 1826.

Houston, J.: Observations on the mucous membrane of the rectum, Dublin Hosp. Rep. *5*:158, 1830.

Kolrausch, C.: Anatomie und Physiologie der Beckenorgane, Leipzig, 1854.

Levy, E.: Anorectal musculature, Am. J. Surg. *34*:141, 1936.

Martin, C. T.: The anorectal line: its clinical significance, Tr. Am. Proct. Soc. *15*:107, 1913.

Milligan, C. T., Morgan, C. W., and Jones, L. E.: Surgical anatomy of the anal canal and the operative treatment of hemorrhoids, Lancet *2*:1119, 1937.

Milligan, E. T. C., and Morgan, C. N.: Surgical anatomy of the anal canal with special reference to fistulae, Lancet *2*:1150, 1934.

Morgan, C. N.: Surgical anatomy of the anal canal and rectum, Postgrad. Med. *22*:287, 1936.

Morgagni, J. G.: Adversaries Anatomica *6*: 111, 1729.

O'Bierne, J.: New Views of the Process of Defecation and Their Application to the Pathogenesis and Treatment of Diseases of the Stomach, Bowels, and Other Organs, Dublin, Hodges and Smith, 1833.

Otis, W. J.: Anatomical researches in the human rectum and a new method of rectal inspection, Leipzig, Veit and Camp, 1887.

Paitre, F., Giraud, D., and Dupret, S.: Pratique anatomo-chirurgicale illustrée. Fasc. II: Région abdominale moyenne et rectum, Paris, Doin, 1935.

Paterson, A.: The form of the rectum, J. Anat. & Physiol. *43*:127, 1909.

Pope, C. E.: Histopathology of anal crypts, Tr. Am. Proct. Soc. *34*:51, 1933.

Stroud, B. B.: On the anatomy of the anus, Ann. Surg. *24*:1, 1896.

Symington, J.: The relations of the peritoneum to the descending colon in the human subject, J. Anat. & Physiol. *26*:530, 1892.

Thompson, P.: Myology of the pelvic floor, Newton, McCorquodale, 1899.

Tucker, C. C., and Hellwig, C. A.: Histopathology of analy crypts, Tr. Am. Proct. Soc. *34*:47, 1933.

Way, S. C., and Memmesheimer, A. The sudoriferous glands, Arch. Dermat. & Syph. *38*:373, 1938.

Wilder, F.: Anal intermuscular septum, Brit. J. Surg. *36*:279, 1949.

ENDOPELVIC FASCIA

Cameron, J.: The fascia of the pelvis, J. Anat. & Physiol. *42*:112, 1907.

Cuneo, B., and Veau, V.: De la signification morphologique des aponeuroses perivesicales, J. Anat. et Physiol. *35*:235, 1899.

Curtis, A. H., Anson, B. J., and Beaton, L. E.: Anatomy of the subperitoneal tissues and ligamentous structures in relation to surgery of the female pelvic viscera, Surg., Gynec. & Obst. *70*:643, 1940.

Denonvilliers, C. P.: Anatomie du perinée, Bull. et mém. Soc. anat. Paris *2*:105, 1836.

Derry, D. E.: On the real nature of the so-called "pelvic fascia," J. Anat. & Physiol. *42*:97, 1907.

Gallaudet, B.: A Description of the Planes of Fasciae of the Human Body with Special Reference to the Fasciae of the Abdomen, Pelvis, and Perineum, New York, Columbia Univ. Press, 1931.

Gorsch, R.: Proctologic considerations of the perineopelvic spaces, Am. J. Surg. *85*:556, 1953.

Hayes, M.: Abdominopelvic fasciae, Am. J. Anat. *87*:119, 1904.

Mackenrodt, A.: Über die Ursachen der normalen und pathologischen Lagen der Uterus, Arch. f. Gynäk. *48*:393, 1895.

Paterson, A.: The mechanical support of the pelvic viscera, Brit. M. J. *2*:1701, 1906.

Reinhold, P.: Contribution à l'étude des recidives postopératoires du cancer rectal, Doctoral thesis, 1924.

Trimpi, H. D., and Bacon, H. E.: Successful nonsurgical reperitonealization of the pelvic floor following radical excision for cancer of rectum, J. Geriatrics *3*:589, 1955.

Sauer, I., and Bacon, H. E.: A new approach for excision of carcinoma of the lower portion of the rectum and anal canal, Surg., Gynec. & Obst. *95*:229, 1952.

Smith, G.: Studies in the anatomy of the pelvis, with special reference to the fasciae and visceral supports. Part II. The rectovesical septum, J. Anat. & Physiol. *42*:198, 1908.

Stoney, R. A.: Anatomy of the visceral pelvic fascia, J. Anat. & Physiol. *38*:438, 1904.

Thompson, P.: On the arrangement of the fasciae of the pelvis and their relationship to the levator ani, J. Anat. & Physiol. *35*:127, 1901.

Tobin, C. E., and Benjamin, J. A.: Anatomical and surgical restudy of the Denonvillier's fascia, Surg., Gynec. & Obst. *80*:373, 1945.

Tobin, C., Benjamin, J. A., and Wells, J. C.: Continuity of the fasciae lining the abdomen, pelvis, and spermatic cord, Surg., Gynec., & Obst. *83*:575, 1946.

Uhlenhuth, E.: Fasciae and subperitoneal fascial spaces of the male pelvic cavity, Bull. School Med. Univ. Maryland *36*:60, 1951.

Uhlenhuth, E., Day, E., Smith, R., and Middleton, E. B.: The visceral endopelvic fascia and hypogastric sheath, Surg., Gynec. & Obst. *86*:9, 1948.

Uhlenhuth, E., Wolfe, W. M., Smith, E. M., and Middleton, E. B.: The rectogenital septum, Surg., Gynec. & Obst. *86*:148, 1948.

Waldeyer, H.: Lehrbuch der topographischen Anatomie, Jossel G. *2*:552, 1899.

Wesson, M. B.: Development and surgical importance of the rectourethralis muscle and Denonvilliers' fascia, J. Urol. *8*:339, 1922.

PERINEOPELVIC SPACES

Brick, J. C.: Fistula in the posterior commissure, Tr. Am. Proct. Soc. *11*:80, 1909.

Courtney, H.: Posterior subsphincteric space, its relation to posterior horseshoe fistula, Surg., Gynec. & Obst. *89*:222, 1949.

——: The posterior levator space, its relation to postanal infection, Tr. Am. Proct. Soc. *45*:450, 1946.

——: Superior sphincteric space, Am. J. Surg. *75*:371, 1948.

Gabriel, W. G.: The Principles and Practice of Rectal Surgery, ed. 4, Springfield, Thomas, 1948.

Milligan, E. T.: Surgical anatomy and disorders of the perianal space, Proc. Roy. Soc. Med. *36*:365, 1943.

Morgan, C. N.: Surgical Anatomy of ischiorectal space, President's Address, Proc. Roy. Soc. Med. *42*:189, 1949.

Patel, M., and Viannay, C.: Topographie de la cavité retrorectale, Lyon méd. *102*:1173, 1904.

OTHER PELVIC STRUCTURES

Bacon, H. E., Dirbas, F., Myers, T. B., and de Leon, P.: Extensive lymphadenectomy and high ligation of the inferior mesenteric artery for carcinoma of the left colon and rectum, Dis. Colon & Rectum *1*:457, 1958.

Cattell, R. B., and Swinton, N. W.: One stage abdominoperineal operation for cancer of the rectum, Dis. Colon & Rectum *2*:253, 1959.

Keyes, H. B.: Carcinoma of the rectum and rectosigmoid: ligation of the internal iliac arteries, Surg., Gynec. & Obst. *67*:512, 1938.

McGregor, R. A.: Ligation of the hypogastric arteries in combined abdominoperineal surgery, Dis. Colon & Rectum *2*:166, 1959.

Remington, J. H.: Prevention of ureteral injury in surgery of the pelvic colon, Dis. Colon & Rectum *2*:340, 1959.

Schaeffer, J. P.: Morris' Human Anatomy, ed. 10, Philadelphia, Blakiston, 1951.

Thorek, P.: Anatomy in Surgery, Philadelphia, Lippincott, 1951.

PERITONEUM

Bochdalek, U.: Über der Peritonealueberzug der Milz und das Ligamentus pleurocolicum, Arch. f. Anat. u. Wissensch. Med., 1867.

Broesike, G.: Über intrabdominále Hernien und Bauchfelltaschen, nebst einer Darstellung der Enwicklung peritonealer Formationen, Berlin, Fisher, 1891.

Douglas, J.: Description of the Peritoneum and of That Part of the Membrana Cellularis Which Lies on the Outside, London, 1730.

Durand, G.: Le ligament ilio-ovarian; contribution à létude des ligaments larges, Progres méd., vol. 3, 1895.

Eastman, J. R.: The fetal peritoneal folds of Jonnesco, Surg., Gynec. & Obst. *16*:341, 1913.

Eve, F. S.: A case of strangulated hernia into the fossa intersigmoidea, Brit. M. J. *1*:1195, 1885.

Flint, J. M.: Embryonic bands and membranes about the cecum, Bull. Johns Hopkins Hosp. *23*:302, 1912.

Haen, D.: Ratio Medendi in nosommio Practice, Vienna, Kruchten, 1771.

Henle, F.: Handbuch der systematischen Anatomie des Menschen, Braunschweig, Vieweg, 1855.

Hildebrandt, O.: Grundriss der chirurgisch-topographischen Anatomie, ed. 2, Weisbaden, Bergman, 1900.

Huntington, G. S.: Anatomy of the Peritoneum and Abdominal Cavity, Philadelphia, Lea Bros., 1903.

Hyrtl, H.: Handbuch der topographischen Anatomie, Vienna, Braumuller, 1865.

Husche and Henle, F.: Handbuch der topographischen Anatomie, ed. 7, Vienna, Braumuller, 1882.

Jackson, J. N.: Membranous pericolitis, Surg., Gynec. & Obst. *10*:278, 1909.

Jonnesco, T.: Hernies internes, retropéritoneales, Paris, G. Steinheil, 1890.

——: Anatomie topographique due duodenum et hernies duodenales, Paris, Lecrosnier et Babe, 1889.

Landzent, H.: Über die Hernie retroperitonealis (Treitz) und ihre Beziehungen zue Fossa duodeno-jejunalis, Med. Ztschr. *30*:350, 1894.

Lane, W.: The kinks which may develop in our drainage system in chronic intestinal stasis, Brit. M. J. *1*:913, 1911.

Lockwood, C. B., and Rolleston, L.: On the fossae around the cecum, J. Anat. & Physiol. *26*:130, 1892.

Longyear, H. W.: Nephrocoloptosis. Kidney and colon suspension by nephrocolic ligament and Gerota's capsule, Surg., Gynec. & Obst. *3*:703, 1906.

Luschka, H.: Über die peritoneale Enthüllinig des Blindarmes und über Fossa ileocecalis, Virchow's Arch. path. Anat. *21*:285, 1861.

Mall, F.: Development of the human intestine and its position in the adult, Bull. Johns Hopkins Hosp. *23*:197, 1898.

Morrison, J.: The anatomy of the right hypochondrium relating especially to operation for gallstones, Brit. M. J. *2*:968, 1904.

Moynihan, G. A.: Retroperitoneal Hernia, ed. 2, London, Baillière, Tindall & Cox, 1906.

Reid, D. E.: Studies in the intestine and peritoneum in the human fetus, J. Anat. & Physiol. *14*:73, 1911.

Retzius, A.: Über des Ligamentum pelviprostaticum oder den Apparat durch welchen die Harnblase, die Prostate un die Harnrohre an der unteren Beckenoffnung Befestigt sind, Arch. f. Anat., Physiol. und Wissensch. Med. 1849.

Sandifort, E.: Tabulae intestini duodeni, Lugauni Bataviorum, Eyk, 1780.

Schott, L.: Beiträge zur Anatomie der Fossa ileocecalis, Wchnbl. d. kk. Gesell. d. Aerzte in Wien *18*:345, 1862.

Tarenentzky, F. G.: Beiträge zur Anatomie des Darmkanals, Mem. Acad. de St. Petersburg, 1881.

Tuffier, T.: Etude sur le cecum et les hernies, Arch. gén. méd. *1*:641, 1887.

Waldeyer, H.: Hernia, retroperitoneale nebst Bemerkungen zur Anatomie des Peritoneums, Breslau, Jungfer, 1808.

BLOOD SUPPLY

Archibald, E. J.: Operative treatment of cancer of the rectum, J.A.M.A. *50*:573, 1908.

Bacon, H. E.: Résumé of experimental studies in proctology in the Graduate and Temple University Hospitals, Read Before the Proctologic Society of the Graduate School, Feb. 21, 1934.

Bacon, H. E., Ross, S. T., and Recio, P. M.: Proctology, Philadelphia, Lippincott, 1956.

Bacon, H. E., and Smith, C. H.: The arterial supply of the distal colon pertinent to abdominoperineal proctosigmoidectomy with preservation of the sphincter mechanism, Ann. Surg. *127*:28, 1934.

Basmajian, J. V.: Main arteries of the large intestine, Surg., Gynec. & Obst. *101*:585, 1955.

Cole, W. H., Packard, D., and Southwick, H. W.: Carcinoma of the colon with special reference to prevention of recurrence, J.A.M.A. *155*:1549, 1954.

Cruz, E. P., McDonald, G. O., and Cole, W. H.: Prophylactic treatment of cancer, Surgery *40*:291, 1956.

Drummond, H.: Some points relating to the surgical anatomy of the arterial supply of the large intestine, Proc. Roy. Soc. Med. *7*: 185, 1913.

——: The arterial supply of the rectum and pelvic colon, Brit. J. Surg. *1*:667, 1914.

Economou, S. G., Mzarek, R., Southwick, H., McDonald, G. O., Slaughter, D., and Cole, W. H.: Prophylactic measures in the spread of carcinoma of the colon and rectum, Dis. Colon & Rectum *2*:98, 1959.

Goligher, J. C.: Blood supply of sigmoid colon and rectum, Brit. J. Surg. *37*:157, 1947.

Hartman, H.: Some considerations upon high amputation of the rectum, Ann. Surg. *50*: 1091, 1909.

Molliere, D.: Traité du rectum, Paris, Masson, 1878.

Pope, C. E., and Buie, L. A.: A description of the arterial blood supply of the sigmoid, rectosigmoid, and rectum, S. Clin. North America *9*:957, 1929.

Rankin, F. W., and Graham, S. A.: Cancer of the Colon and Rectum, ed. 2, Springfield, Thomas, 1950.

Reuther, T. F.: The values and anastomoses of the hemorrhoidal and related veins, Am. J. Surg. *49*:326, 1940.

Riolan, J., Jr.: Manual anatomique et pathologique au abrégé de toute l'anatomie, Nouv. ed. Lyon, 1672.

Robillard, G. L., and Shapiro, A. L.: Variational anatomy of the middle colic artery, its significance in gastric and colonic surgery, J. Internat. Coll. Surgeons *10*:157, 1947.

Rubesch, R.: Über die Vermeidung der Darmgangrän bei Rektumoperationen, Beitr. klin. Chir. *67*:480, 1910.

Singleton, A. O.: The blood supply of the large bowel with reference to resection, Surgery *14*:328, 1943.

Steward, J. A., and Rankin, F. W.: Blood supply of the large intestine; its surgical considerations, Arch. Surg. *26*:843, 1933.

Sudeck, P.: Über Gefässversorgung des Mastdarms in Hinicht auf die operative Gangrän, München. med. Wchnschr. *54*:1314, 1907.

Sunderland, S.: Blood supply of the distal colon, Australian & New Zealand J. Surg. *11*: 253, 1942.

Thorek, P.: Anatomy in Surgery, Philadelphia, Lippincott, 1951.

LYMPHATIC DRAINAGE

Bacon, H. E., and Sauer, I.: Surgical treatment of cancer of the lower bowel, Cancer *3*: 773, 1950.

Bacon, H. E., and Trimpi, H. D.: Rectal cancer: inferior mesenteric regional lymph node dissection with ligation of the inferior mesenteric artery at its origin; report of 261 cases, West. J. Surg. *63*:181, 1955.

Cloquet, J.: Recherches anatomiques sur les hernies de l'abdomen, Paris, Meqnignon Marois, 1817.

Coller, F. A., Kay, E. B., and McIntire, R. C.: Regional metastasis of carcinoma of rectum, Surgery *8*:294, 1940.

Cuneo, B., and Marcille, M.: Lymphatiques iliaques, Bull. et mém. Soc. anat. Paris *12*: 281, 1901.

D'Allaines, F., Leroy, A., and Dubost, C.: Traitement Chirurigical du Cancer du Rectum, Paris, Flammarion, 1946.

Delamere, G.: The Lymphatics, Chicago, Keener, 1904.

Drinker, C. K. and Field, M. E.: Lymphatics, Lymph and Tissue Fluid, Baltimore, Williams & Wilkins, 1933.

Dukes, C. E.: The spread of cancer of the rectum, Brit. J. Surg. *17*:643, 1930.

Economou, S. G., Mzarek, R., Southwick, H., McDonald, G. O., Slaughter, D., and Cole, W. H.: Prophylactic measures in the spread of carcinoma of the colon and rectum, Dis. Colon & Rectum *2*:98, 1959.

Gerota, D.: Die Lymphgefässe des Rektums und des Anus, Arch. f. Anat. u Physiol. Anat. *14*:240, 1895.

——: Über die Lymphgefässe und die Lymphdrüsen der Nabelgegend und der Harnblase, Anat. Anz. *12*:89, 1896.

Gilchrist, R. K.: Lymphatic spread of carcinoma of the colon, Dis. Colon & Rectum *2*:69, 1959.

Glaudier, H.: Traitement du cancer du rectum, Soc. Chir. Paris, Sem. Med. Par. *16*: 133, 1896.

Grinnell, R. S.: Lymphatic and venous spread of carcinoma of rectum, Ann. Surg. *116*: 200, 1942.

——: The spread of carcinoma of the colon and rectum, Cancer *3*:641, 1950.

Hochenegg, J.: Bestrebungen zur chirurgischen Behandlungen des Mastdamkrebses Operierten, Wien med. Wchnschr. *5*:59, 1909.

Jackson, R. B.: Carcinoma of the colon; avenues of spread and methods of preventing recurrence, Dis. Colon & Rectum *1*:186, 1958.

Jamieson, J. K.: Lymphatics of the colon, Proc. Roy. Soc. Med. *2*:149, 1907.

Jamieson, J. K., and Dobson, J. F.: Lymphatics of the colon, Ann. Surg. *50*:1077, 1909.

Looney, W. W.: Lymphatic distribution of the colon and rectum, Am. J. Surg. *46*:143, 1939.

Marcille, M.: Lymphatiques et ganglions iliopelviens, Paris, Thesis, 1909.

Mascagni, P.: Vasorum lymyhaticorum corporis humani historia et ichonographia, Senis, Carli, 1787.

McElwain, J., Bacon, H. E., and Trimpi, H. D.: Lymph node metastasis, Surgery *35*: 513, 1954.

McKittrick, L. S.: Resection of the colon for carcinoma, Dis. Colon & Rectum *2*:123, 1959.

Mondor, H.: Contribution à l'étude au cancer du rectum, Paris, Thesis, 1914.

Nesselrod, J. P.: An anatomic restudy of the pelvic lymphatics, Ann. Surg. *104*:905, 1936.

Oliviera, E.: Observacas sobre os linfaticos anoretais, These, Rio de Janeiro, 1944.

Peham, H., and Amreich, H.: Gynecologische Operationslehre, Berlin, S. Karger, 1930.

Poirier, P., and Charpy, A.: Traité d'anatomie humaine, Paris, Masson, 1889.

Poirier, P., Cuneo, B., and Delamere, G.: The Lymphatics, London, Constable, 1913.

Quenu, E.: Vaisseaux lymphatiques de l'anus, Bull. Soc. anat. Paris *68*:399, 1893.

Reinhold, P.: Contribution à l'étude des recidives postopératoires du cancer rectal, Doct. Thesis, 1924.

Reybard, J. F.: Mémoire sur une tumuer cancéreuse affectant l'illiaque du colon, Bull. Acad. méd. Paris *9*:1031, 1844.

Rosi, P. A.: Selection of operations for carcinomas of the colon, S. Clin. North America *34*:221, 1954.

Rouviere, H.: Anatomie des lymphatiques de l'homme, Paris, Masson, 1932.

Sauer, I., and Bacon, H. E.: A new approach for excision of carcinoma of the lower portion of the rectum and anal canal, Surg., Gynec. & Obst. *95*:229, 1952.

Sauer, I., and Bacon, H. E.: Influence of lateral spread of cancer of rectum on radicability, Am. J. Surg. *31*:111, 1951.

Schoenbauer, L., and Pfab, B.: Über Rektum-Karcinom, Wien. med. Wchnschr. *76*:1295, 1929.

Semba, Y.: Anatomische Untersuchungen über das Lympgefässysteme des Rektum, mit besonderer Berucksichtigung der Metastasenbildung des Rektumkrebes, Arch. klin. Chir. *149*:336, 1928.

Spalteholz, W. A.: Method for Clearing of Human and Animal Specimens, Leipzig, S. Herzel, 1911.

Villemin, F., Huard, P., and Montague, M.: Recherches anatomiques sur les lymphatiques du rectum et de l'annus, leur applications dans le traitment chirurgicale du cancer, Rev. chir. Paris *63*:39, 1925.

Von Appalger, B., and Nietsche, L.: Ergebnisse und Erfahrungen mit der Chirurgischen Therapye des Mastdarmkrebses, Arch. klin. Chir. *203*:159, 1949.

Westheus, H.: Die pathologisch-anatomischen Grundlagen der Chirurgie des Rektum Karzinoms, Leipzig, Thieme, 1934.

NERVE SUPPLY

Abel, A. L.: The surgery of the sympathetic nervous system, Post-Grad. Surg. *11*:3112, 1936.

Goligher, J. C., and Hughes, E. S. R.: Sensibility of rectum and colon; its role in mechanism of anal incontinence, Lancet *1*:543, 1951.

Hallenbeck, G. A.: Anterior resection and "pull-through" procedure for cancer of the rectum and rectosigmoid, Dis. Colon & Rectum *2*:117, 1959.

Klinge, F. W.: Motor functions of the cat's colon following excision of Auerbach's plexus, Ann. Surg. *136*:162, 1952.

Labate, J. S.: The surgical anatomy of the superior hypogastric plexus, Surg., Gynec. & Obst. *67*:199, 1938.

Langley, J. N., and Anderson, H.: On the innervation of the pelvis and the adjoining viscera, J. Physiol. *18*:67, 1895.

Laterjet, A., and Bonnett, B.: Le plexus hypogastrique chez l'homme, Lyon chir. *9*:619, 1933.

Laux, G.: Contribution à l'étude anatomique des sympathétiques pelviens: déductions chirurgicales, Lyons, Freres et Riou, 1927.

McCrea, L. E., and Kimmel, D. L.: The importance of nerve supply of the urinary bladder in surgery of the rectosigmoid, J. Internat. Coll. Surgeons *17*:651, 1952.

Oppenheimer, M. J., and Glyer, N. M.: Effect of elevated metabolism on rate of intestinal contractions, Am. J. Digest. Dis. *8*:471, 1941.

Reuther, T. F.: Nerves of the anorectal region, Tr. Am. Proct. Soc. *41*:202, 1940.

Recio, P. M., and Oppenheimer, M. J.: Investigation into the effects of altered acid-base equilibrium upon the motility of the colon, Am. J. Surg. *86*:591, 1953.

Schlitt, R. J., McNally, J. J., and Hinton, J. W.: Response of the distal colon to external stimuli, Surg., Gynec. & Obst. *92*:223, 1951.

Spiegel, E. A., Weston, K., and Oppenheimer, M. J.: Postmotor foci influencing the gastrointestinal tract and their descending pathways, Neuropath. & Exper. Neurol. *2*:45, 1943.

Telford, E. D., and Stafford, J. S.: The anatomic nerve supply of the distal colon: an anatomical and clinical study, Brit. M. J. *1*: 572, 1932.

Wells, J. A., Mercer, T. H., Gray, J. S., and Ivy, A. C.: Motor innervation of the colon, Am. J. Physiol. *138*:83, 1942.

White, J. C.: Progress in surgery of the autonomic nervous system, Surgery *23*:834, 1948.

PHYSIOLOGY

Alvarez, W. C.: Mechanics of the Digestive Tract, New York, Hoeber, 1922.

Alvarez, W. C., and Starkweather, E.: The metabolic gradient underlying colonic peristalsis, Am. J. Physiol. *47*:293, 1918.

Bayliss, W. M., and Starling, E. H.: Movements and innervation of the large intestine, J. Physiol. *26*:107, 1900.

Frankl-Hockwart, L. V., and Frolich, A.: Über Tonus und Innervation der Sphinkteren des Anus, Arch. f. d. ges. Physiol. *81*: 420, 1900.

Howell, W. H.: Textbook of Physiology, ed. 8, Philadelphia, Saunders, 1933.

Kastle und Bruegal: Die Bewegungsvorgange des menschlichen Dünn- und Dickdarmes während der Verdauung auf Grund röntgenographischer und röntgenkinomatographischer Untersuchungen, München. med. Wchnschr. *59*:446, 1912.

Kohn, L. W.: Diseases of Digestive System, vol. 1, Philadelphia, Davis, 1930.

Langley, J. N., and Anderson, H. K.: On the innervation of the pelvic and adjoining viscera, J. Physiol. *18*:67, 1895.

Lynch, J., and Felsen, J.: Tumors of the Rectum and Colon, New York, Hoeber, 1925.

O'Beirne, J.: New Views of the Process of Defecation, Dublin, Hodges & Smith, 1833.

Sunderland, F. W., and Boerner, F.: Normal Values in Clinical Medicine, Philadelphia, Saunders, 1949.

Todd, J. C., and Sanford, A. H.: Clinical Diagnosis by Laboratory Methods, ed. 11, Philadelphia, Saunders, 1948.

Additional Reference:

Best, C. H., and Taylor, N. B.: The Physiological Basis of Medical Practice, ed. 5, Baltimore, Williams & Wilkins, 1950.

Index